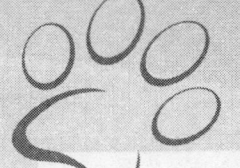

Veterinary Practice

A Manual

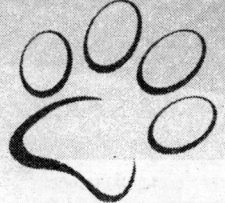

Veterinary Practice

A Manual

HVS Chauhan

BVSc, MVSc, (Gold Medalist) Jabalpur University, PhD (Honours)
Punjab Agricultural University, PD Perth, Australia, FIAVP (New Delhi)
Veterinary Consultant, Nandini Veterinary Hospital, Surat
Retd Dean (Vet. Faculty) Indira Gandhi Agricultural University, Raipur, (6 ½ years)
Head, Pathology, Birsa Agricultural University, Ranchi (16 years)
Head, Dvn. Avian Diseases IVRI, Izzatnagar
Associate Professor, Haryana Agricultural University, Hissar
Ex Editor, Indian J. Vet. Path (1978 onward)
Ex Associate Editor, Indian J. Animal Sci (ICAR)
Awards: Dr Rajendra Prasad Award (ICAR), Indira Gandhi Award, (Government of India)
GA Shastri Award (Indian Vet. Assoc.) Distinguished Leadership Award (USA)
Dr PP Gupta Award (Indian Vet. Path Assoc.)
Colombo Plan Fellowship for PD in Australia
Author of Poultry Diseases Diagnosis and Treatment (4th Edn, 2016) and 7 other books

Hardik Soni

MVSc (Pharma), Private
Pet Clinic, Surat

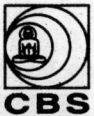

CBS

CBS Publishers & Distributors Pvt Ltd

New Delhi • Bengaluru • Chennai • Kochi • Kolkata • Mumbai
Bhopal • Bhubaneswar • Hyderabad • Jharkhand • Nagpur • Patna • Pune • Uttarakhand • Dhaka (Bangladesh)

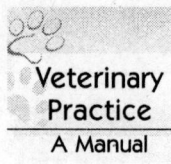

Veterinary Practice
A Manual

ISBN: 978-93-88725-66-8

First Edition: 2020

Published by Satish Kumar Jain and produced by Varun Jain for

CBS Publishers & Distributors Pvt Ltd
4819/XI Prahlad Street, 24 Ansari Road, Daryaganj, New Delhi 110 002, India.
Ph: 23289259, 23266861, 23266867   Fax: 011-23243014   Website: www.cbspd.com
                                                                    e-mail: delhi@cbspd.com; cbspubs@airtelmail.in
Corporate Office: 204 FIE, Industrial Area, Patparganj, Delhi 110 092
Ph: 4934 4934   Fax: 4934 4935   e-mail: publishing@cbspd.com;   publicity@cbspd.com

Branches

- **Bengaluru:** Seema House, 2975, 17th Cross, K.R. Road,
  Banasankari 2nd Stage, Bengaluru 560 070, Karnataka
  Ph: +91-80-26771678/79   Fax: +91-80-26771680   e-mail: bangalore@cbspd.com
- **Chennai:** 7, Subbaraya Street, Shenoy Nagar, Chennai 600 030, Tamil Nadu
  Ph: +91-44-26680620, 26681266   Fax: +91-44-42032115   e-mail: chennai@cbspd.com
- **Kochi:** 42/1325, 1326, Power House Road, Opposite KSEB Power House,
  Ernakulam 682 018, Kochi, Kerala
  Ph: +91-484-4059061-65   Fax: +91-484-4059065   e-mail: kochi@cbspd.com
- **Kolkata:** 6/B, Ground Floor, Rameswar Shaw Road, Kolkata-700 014, West Bengal
  Ph: +91-33-22891126, 22891127, 22891128   e-mail: kolkata@cbspd.com
- **Mumbai:** 83-C, Dr E Moses Road, Worli, Mumbai-400018, Maharashtra
  Ph: +91-22-24902340/41   Fax: +91-22-24902342   e-mail: mumbai@cbspd.com

Representatives

• Bhopal	0-8319310552	• Bhubaneswar	0-9911037372	• Hyderabad	0-9885175004
• Nagpur	0-9421945513	• Patna	0-9334159340	• Pune	0-9623451994
• Dhaka (Bangladesh)	01912-003485	• Jharkhand	0-9811541605	• Uttarakhand	0-9716462459

Printed at: Mudrak, Noida, UP, India

Preface

This book is aimed at providing a practical and result-oriented line of treatment based on my 12 years of experience as Veterinary Consultant, dealing with about 6000 grown up (old) cows, calves and about 700–800 sheep and goats which have been kept on humanitarian grounds at the place I am working. My job is to prevent diseases and deaths of these animals so that it does not cross 0.6% per day. At another campus of my place of work, about 5000 cow calves and buffalo calves and heifers are kept with the same objective. About 500 dairy cows and pregnant animals are also kept to control diseases and mortality. Nandini Veterinary Hospital of our organization deals with about 80–100 cases mostly pets daily and has good indoor facilities.

Most of the new practitioners need, beside theoretical academic knowledge which they get in colleges, a guideline for drugs and practical clinical approach to be successful. This book should be able to help them in terms of practical knowledge.

I have worked as a veterinary doctor since 1959, having worked as Veterinary Assistant Surgeon and later, as a teacher and researcher, and holding positions like Head, Division of Avian Diseases at IVRI, Izzatnagar, and also as Dean of Veterinary College under Indira Gandhi Agricultural University, Raipur for many years. Presently, I am working at Surat Panjrapole cum Nandini Veterinary Hospital as a Consultant Doctor.

I wish to add my long clinical experience and have evaluated selection of about 40 pharmaceutical companies of India listed in the book. A list of various categories of drugs are also given as index for doctors' selection.

Less important or rare diseases have been excluded because the doctors are familiar with them and also to keep the manual within limits. Details of various vaccines and pet food products are also dealt within detail.

A chapter on 'Sure Shots' of homoeopathy deals with homoeopathic medicines which are just wonderful but they should be used under qualified homoeopathic advise.

Statistical information, physiological and clinical parameters, vaccination charts for cattle, sheep, goat, and dog are also included for ready reference.

Another book of mine, *Poultry Diseases, Diagnosis and Treatment* has been published for the last 20 years (presently in 4th edition). Poultry diseases are therefore excluded from this manual.

I hope the doctors will find this book easy for prescription. Please send your suggestions and comments, if any, for further improvement.

HVS Chauhan

Acknowledgements

My hearty thanks to my wife, Shobha Chauhan and my dear son, Anurag Chauhan (presently Head, Department of English and Foreign Languages at Guru Ghasidas Vishwavidyalaya, a Central University) for their unflinching support. My son, Anurag, also typed meticulously the manuscript for this manual inspite of his workload.

Dr Hardik Soni, the co-author, was helpful in updating the portion on canine diseases. My other doctor friends, Dr Vimal Kumar Pandey, Dr Jigar Parekh, and Gelani deserve thanks for their constructive suggestions.

The livestock inspectors working with me in the branches, in particular, Shri Harpal, Gavit, Sagar, Girase, Navneet, Tejas, and Farm Managers, Ambalal Patel and Sharad Bhai deserve special thanks for their help in treatment, preventive measures and vaccinations, etc.

Caution: The readers should be careful about doses and side effects, holding period of products, post-medication and the authors cannot take the responsibility inspite of the utmost care taken in these matters.

HVS Chauhan

Contents

How to Use This Manual

I understand that senior doctors and professors are wise enough and knowledgeable hence they do not need any advise.

For students and new practitioners of suggest to rely more on "Alphabetical Index" of topics/diseases to find out the line of approach/medicines without inconvenience. For example, if you want to know about anthrax look it under 'A' and turn to page 22 to know all about anthrax.

Second suggestion is about "Classified Index of Medicines" This part is essential because if medicine given in the topic/subject are not available in your town or place of work you can find out alternative medicines in this index.

Third, the "Sure Shots of Homoeopathy" are based on my own personal experience and some of them have been mentioned under different topics. These are not final and may not always work hence they should be used exceptionally after consulting a qualified homoeopath.

Last, I have tried my best to be accurate about dose and other particulars, side effects, etc. but I cannot take responsibility about dose, indications, nonindications, side effects reactions, etc. for which the doctor himself should take care and be responsible for consequences.

The manual is like a friend but "not final authority" on topic/disease/line of treatment "To err is human" only God is without error.

I welcome suggestions and your valuable advice in any respect to correct, modify or add to the value of the manual.

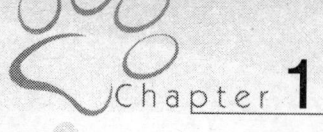

Chapter 1

Calf Management and Health

▨ NEWBORN CALVES

Newborn calves require very special attention for health and survival, they are very weak specially in regards to immunity. Death is most common in 1 month post-delivery.

▨ GENERAL STEPS AFTER BIRTH

1. Take or assess the weight of the calf at birth, higher the weight better chances of survival. Specially in cold season and rainy season:
   - Average weight of healthy cow calf is between 20 and 35 kg
   - Average weight of good buffalo calf 30–40 kg.
2. Take maximum care of calf for 8 hours, feed warm mother's colostrum by natural suckling or if unable to suckle than by feeding bottle.

   Death during 48 hours after birth: Calves which become sick and die within first 48 hours after calving are not likely to die due to infections hence do not switch over to antibiotics unless marked fever is recorded

▨ MORTALITY DURING 48 HOURS AFTER CALVING

Death during first 48 hours after calving are due to:
1. Metabolic cause, mostly hypoglycemia which may be manifested by subnormal body temperature (hypothermia).
2. Congenital diseases.
3. Enterotoxins of toxicogenic *E. coli*, which cause death due to shock by heatstable toxin.

▨ MORTALITY DURING 28 DAYS

First Week Mortality

Causes: Most of the mortality occurs due to immunoglobulin deficiency due to failure of their transfer into body from colostrum *E. coli* infections are most common, less common causes are septicaemia and viral (rotavirus) infections.

Second to Fourth Week Mortality

In this period diarrhoea and pneumonia, naval ill, arthritis may occur due to failure of immunoglobulin transfer from intestines. It can be summerised that most of the diseases in newborn calves occur due to non-transfer of immunoglobulins.

OTHER FACTORS

1. Heat or cold stress: Ideal temperature 31 to 37°C
2. Hypoxia during dystocia
3. Twin born calves
4. Premature birth: Normal gestation in calf (240 days)
5. Congenital defects
6. Nutritional deficiency from mother: Iodine, copper, cobalt, manganese, vitamin D and vitamin A can increase calf mortality
7. Poor mothering instinct: Hence cannot suck colostrum.

NORMAL CALF MORTALITY

Normal calf mortality varies from country to country and also from climatic factors (more in hot climate) and breed to breed (more in exotic breeds like Holsteins, slightly less in Jerseys and lesser still in Indian breeds like Sahiwal, Gir, Sindhi, Kankrej, etc.). In USA, inspite of ideal livestock management mortality varies from 2 to 60%. (Radostis et al 2009, Veterinary Preventive Medicine, 128) and 6.8 to 11.9% in England and south Scotland (White and Jordan vety Prev. Med, 200, first Indian ed.). in India cow calf mortality is 42.8% (Malhotra and Parmar, 2007, Indian Vet J. 2007, 83:607–9) in organized farms. In calves below 1 month mortality in India is 51.8% (Radhakrishnan KV, 2007, Indian Vet J. 84:537–9).

Causes are: Digestive diseases/enteritis (17.7%)
Respiratory diseases (15.4%)
Septicaemis 21.5%
Miscellaneous causes 45.4%

STEPS FOR REDUCING CALF MORTALITY

1. Let the calf suckle colostrum from mother. If there is any reason (dystocia, milk fever, death of mother) feed colostrum with milk bottle. The calf must get warm colostrum as early as possible after delivery and in any case before 8 hours after birth.
2. Warm (body temperature) colostrum results in closure of oesophageal grove which takes it into abomasum. If cold colostrum is fed it will go into rumen which is unable to digest milk. The milk in rumen is putrified by the contaminated bacteria most commonly *E. coli*. Undigested milk and *E. coli*. produce diarrhoea called "white scours" which may kill the calf.
   Immunoglobulins of colostrum are also lost through diarrhoic faeces which almost always results in death inspite of antibiotics therapy.
3. Provide good ventilation and warmroom (in winter).
4. The cut end of umbilicus is closed with a ligature, preferably suture material) and dressed liberally with tincture of iodine or broad-spectrum antibiotic ointment. Dressing may be repeated for a few days.
5. After feeding on colostrum give half spoonful of pulsatilla 200 (homoepathic medicine) mixed with a little water, once in a day for easy digestion and stimulation of appetite.
6. Keep sanitized and preferably medicated water for calves in case they drink. For example "chlortech" (vetcare) which is 2.5 times more potent than chlorine. It is added at the rate of 1 ml per litre water. It kills bacteria, viruses and protozoa.

'Isochlor' (polchem product). It effectively kills bacteria, fungi, protozoa and virus. 1 tablet is to be dissolved in 1000 litre of water, chlorine based sanitiser.

7. Wash the calf pen first with a detergent to scrub off deposits which prevent disinfection. For disinfection of calf pen follow the instructions of marketed or branded disinfectants. Formalin is very effective disinfectant which may be used as 3 to 5% solution in water to disinfect floor, tiled walls and utensils.

8. Lime powder may be sprinkled at the rate of 4 to 7 kg per 100 sq. feet. It generates heat and kills parasite eggs, coccidia and bacteria. Lime is used for open yard having dust and clay.

9. Other branded disinfectants can also be used such as Medichlor S, Dettol, Virkon -S (Pfizer), Kohrsolin (Virbac), Glufort (Zydus), Chlorosol (Intervet), etc.

10. Chlorasol (Intervet) contains N chloro-para-toluene-sulfonamide and is a very good disinfectant which kills wide range of bacteria, viruses, and fungi from floors and even from equipments, transport vehicles, machinery, etc. It is used at the dose rate of 3 g per litre of water.

11. "Isochlor"– Isochlor is available as 5 g tablets. It is dissolved at the rate of 5 g in 1000 litres of water in drinking water (polchem lab, pvt. ltd.)

12. Infection of umbilicus occurs soon after birth due to mixed infection of *E. coli*, *Proteus sp.*, *Staphylococcus sp.*, etc which, if neglected, will result in bacteraemia/ septicaemia and localization in joints (arthritis), fever of unknown origin, meninges (meningitis), eyes (ophthalmitis). Umbilical infection (omphalitis) commonly occurs at 2–5 days after birth and is very problematic, persisting for several weeks. Ligation of umbilicus soon after birth and liberal and daily painting of umbilicus with tincture of iodine is usually done in India. The results of modern research show that 7% iodine should be used for the umbilicus. Second best choice is application of Chlorhexidine (Indian preparation, Dermichlor of Vetoquinol India Animal Health or Chlor Hexol of Neospark Drugs and Chemicsls, 50 and 100 ml bottles).

13. Drinking water of calves should not be hard. It should be pure, cool and 1 tablet of 'Klengard' should be added per 250 litres of drinking water for a week or for 15 days. (container of 5 tablets, Intas Animal Health)

14. At the onset of fever or diarrhea, give Quinintas daily for 3–5 days. Intalyte (oral) of Intas Animal Health may also be given (20 g/litre of water)

▣ EFFECT OF HEAT AND HUMIDITY

Newborn calves should be protected from excessive heat and cold. Both have killer effect even without any other diseases. In such hot weather use following medicines.

1. Replina—available as 1 kg pack. It is mixed in drinking water at the rate of 1 g in 2 litres water. It is a modern preparation containing glycine and protein hydrolysate, sodium bicarbonate, sodium citrate, magnisium chloride, calcium lactate and vitamin C (TTK product).

2. Heat combination of homoepathic medicines:
   - Glonoine 6–5 ml
   - Selenium 6–5 ml
   - Coca 6–5 ml
   - Naja 30–5 ml

These medicines are mixed and given by mouth at the rate of about 8–10 drops per calf or they may be given in drinking water.

3. Glonoine 6 or 30—liquid 1 dram
   1–3 drops of this homoepathic medicine is a perfect medicine for heat stress (repeat 2–3 times if required). It cures heat stroke in humans.
4. Vitamin C/ascorbic acid—available as injection or tablets. Higher doses—about twice the normal dose.
5. Glucaboost liquid orally to meet out high calory requirement (natural remedies). The calves under the effect of heat will pant with mouth open (as in dogs). Dose for cattle: 200 ml once daily. It is gluconeogenic solution.

PROTECTION FROM COLD AND HYPOTHERMIA

Weak calves or even normal calves exposed to severe cold may suffer from hypothermia. Newborn calves on first day may have normal body temperature of 13°C or 55 to 59° F. To save them from hypothermia.
1. Keep them in sunlight.
2. Give warm dextrose saline injection mixed with following medicines. I use this mixture by intraperitoneal method which gives immediate response. The recumbent calf sits in about 15–20 minutes after injection and then starts eating after 20–30 minutes.
   - Dextrose saline (10% or or preferably 25%) 100 to 200 ml
   - Vitamin B complex (like Tribivet or Hitek inj.) 10 ml
   - Tonophosphan 10–20 ml
   - Perinorm injection 2 ml
   - Kepkal injection 3 to 4 ml
   - Napler injection 5 ml

All these injectables are mixed in the bottle of dextrose than the bottle of the injectable mixture is heated to make it luke warm (around 40°C) in water bath to avoid direct heating. I use induction heater with water bath. Intraperitoneal injection is given preferably in front of ischium bone with taking precaution not to puncture any abdominal organ or intestine. This is to be used for critical cases otherwise injection of warm dextrose saline or Mifex inj. Or calcium boro gluconate (CBG) by IV route may be adopted.

I also allow the calf to lick "Ruchiboost" a sweet, honey-based appetizer. Intraperitoneal method given here is a non-traditional method and may be used only after written consent of the owner to save a critically serious animal which has hardly any chances of survival or revival as in case of ICU patients in human beings.

This treatment may be repeated if necessary till complete recovery under written consent of the owner.

TEMPERATURE HUMIDITY INDEX (THI) AN EYE OPENER

In general perception that, it is the high environmental temperature (ET) only results into heat stress. Yes, to the extent it is true. But even comparatively low environmental temperature with high humidity may produce much severe stress than only high environmental temperature. The same can be explained by THI furnished below. Temperature with high and low humidity leads to stress, even at low temperature with high humidity animals suffer from stress.

Signs of Heat Stress
- Daily feed intake decreases subclinical rumen acidosis
- Water intake increases blood flow to internal organs decreases but increases in skin
- Respiration rate increases, reproductive performance decreases
- Milk production decreases, decreased levels of blood biocarbonate
- Acute health problems, significant drop in pregnancy rate
- High incidence of abortions, death loss increases
- Decreases saliva production
- Increased drooling of saliva.

▨ MILK REPLACER
Milk replacer is to be fed to calves which have lost their mother or if the cow is sick. Calf replacer may be fed at the rate of 200 g to substitute a litre of cow milk:
- Wheat 8 kg
- Fish meal 12 kg
- Dry milk powder 16 kg
- Linseed meal 40 kg
- Coconut oil 7 kg
- Linseed oil or Ricebran oil 3 kg
- Citric acid 1.4 kg
- Molases 8 kg
- Mineral mixture 3 kg
- Butyric acid 0.60 litres
- Antibiotic mix (such as tetracycline WSPVET of MSD animal health 300 g
- Rovimix (vitamin A, B_2, D_3 and E).

Rate of Feeding Milk Replacer
Schedule of feeding milk replacer diet

Age of (days)	Live wt. (kg)	Milk/day (kg)	Milk replacer (g)
1–5	–	Colostrum 1.0 to 1.5	–
6–14		2	
15–18		2.0	50
19–22		Minus ½ kg[a]	100
23–26		Minus 1.0 kg	300
31–34		Minus 2.0 kg	400
	40	1.0	500
	45	1.0	550
	50	1.0	600
	55	1.0	650
	60	1.0	700
	65	1.0	750
	70	1.0	800
	75	1.0	850
	80	1.0	900
	85	1.0	950
	90	1.0	1000

■ CALF MILK REPLACER 2

If preparation of above calf replacer looks difficult to prepare then use "quickrumi" a product of Zydus company which provides alternate source of calf nutrition which increases glucose available through BHBA, increases development of rumen and allows quicker conversion of solid diet. It reduces weaning age and prevents calf diarrhoea. It is available in 100 g and 500 g packs.

Dosage

Age of calf	Oral dose per day
10–30 days	15 g
1–2 months	20 g
2–3 months	25 g
Above 3 months	30 g

Milk Feeding Bottle

Weak calves, which cannot suckle milk of mother can be artificially fed milk by special calf milk bottle. "Glucaboost" Liquid Energy Booster of Natural Remedies Pvt. ltd. can be fed at recommended dose. Bivinal plus (Alembic) or Belamyl (Zydus) can be injected deep intramuscularly daily for about 1 week at the rate of 0.25 to 0.5 ml, twice a day. If the calf is having muscular weakness inject neuroxine IM or IV at the dose rate of 2–3 ml.

Another product which we use to improve metabolism and provide energy is oral feeding of "vigest" (Bayer product) vigest is fed to calves at dose rate of 30 to 60 ml. Another drug containing polypeptides amino acid, B group of vitamins, iron, magnesium, dextrose and electrolytes can be used.

Immunoglobulin Injections

The senior author of this book prepares and uses purified immunoglobulins at the dose rate of 1.5 to 2.5 g as subcutaneous injection which is extremely useful injection. Its results are obtained with almost no requirement of costly antibiotics or antidiarrhoeal or anti pneumonia drugs if it is injected as early as possible after birth or even in older calves below 6 months age.

This injection is being used by the senior author for the last about 7–8 years without side effects or reaction. It is cheap hardly costing ₹ 50 for one injection which protects against all bacterial diseases for not less than 3 to 4 months but injection needs patenting. If a colostrums deprived calf is saved by antibiotic and other treatments there is very little chance of the calf surviving after 3 months of age.

Loss of Appetite

The calf may not drink milk or may become off feed. This is a serious problem because of weak constitution of calf, for such condition following steps should be taken.

Take temperature: There may be fever which may be due to bacterial infection, for this give antibiotics depending on symptoms (septicaemia, pneumonia, diarrhoea, etc.). Long-acting (LA) (long-acting—for 3 days) antibiotics such as Enromycin LA for 3 to 4 days:

- Chloramphenicol 50 mg/kg orally or IM inj.

- Ciprofloxacin 5–15 mg/kg po, SC or IM BID
- Cipro TZ 5–10 mg/kg IM, IV, SC

In case of no fever:

1. Give injection of perinorm @ 0.5 mg/kg BW by IM route or metoclopramide injection
2. Give Pulsatilla 200 – a homoeopathic liquid ½ tea spoonful once or twice daily.
3. 'Ruchi Boost'—Honey-based appetizer 15 g for 2–3 days. This is applied on lips which is licked by the animal (Product of VanVet Pvt. Ltd. info@vanvet.co.in)

◼ DISEASES OF CALVES (NEWBORN)

Calves are most susceptible to infections and death before 2 weeks of age, particularly diarrhoea and septicaemia. According to survey of many farms in USA by the US department of *agriculture*, 40% calves fail to absorb immunoglobulins from colostrum.

Assisted natural feeding of colostrum by calf may be adopted or about 2 litres of colostrum may be milked out and fed warm to calf. Then the calf is left with mother for 24 hours or bottle feeding of colostrum (warm) at every 12 hours for 48 hours is adopted.

Severe Cold and Hypothermia

Severe cold resulting in hypothermia, very low body temperature below 98° F which is sometimes fatal. Hypothermia in calves or heifer may occur in two seasons:

1. Severe cold (winter)
2. Incessant rains + wind (rainy season)

Due to shortage of energy the metabolism goes to negative side. To prevent this:

1. Use hot air blower (heavy duty) during night
2. Protect animals from direct cold winds or showers by plastic or asbestos sheets.
3. Give jaggary, ginger powder and some oil mixed together to provide energy (about 150 g + 10 g + 30–50 ml).
4. Give "Glucaboost" or "vigest" about 30–50 ml morning and evening (orally).
5. Intraperitoneal injection of combination of drugs (Dextrose 20–25% + B complex such as Tribivet plain or Tribivet M + Tonophosphan 10–15 ml or Urimin or Lyphos vet 15 ml or Napler 12–15 ml). This combination must be heated in water bath to about 40°C + perinorm 2 ml to promote normal stomach and intestinal motility. Also give Ruchi boost paste by mouth for appetite generation (Product of VanVet Pharma, phone: 9375046501) for 1–2 days. It is extremely good.
6. Orally "Ruchiboost" or feed fast gel 30 g (product of Brovet, animal healthcare, Navsari, Gujarat) may be given to stimulate appetite, morning and evening.

In recent times I got success in saving dozens of hypothermic (temperature range 92 to 98 degree celcius) plus severe anaemia (below 7g/dl) afflicted calves by intraperitoneal injections of colostrum mixed with 5–6 more ingredients.

High Environment Temperature

Causes of hyperthermia in particular species of animals, buffaloes are more affected by high environmental temperature. Cows are more affected than heifers. In buffaloes I have seen calves panting like dogs with mouth open and tongue partly protruding from mouth. Common causes of hyperthermia also include, some type of poisioning or drugs. For example, ergot poisoning, levamisol overdose, iodine toxicity, strychnine toxicity, etc.

Diagnosis

Rectal temperature above 39.5°C or 103°F, breathing rate becomes high, sweating, salivation, restlessness followed by dullness. Liking for cool-shaded place temperature more than 8°F above normal temperature is fatal. Prolonged hyperthermia may cause infertility. Clotting of blood is slow.

Treatment

1. Giving cool or chilled water.
2. Shower with water.
3. Use of fans and good ventilation (exhaust fans).
4. Provide more vitamin C or injections of high doses.

Chapter 2

Fever or Pyrexia

Causes

1. Septicaemia
2. Pyogenic or other infections
3. Pyrexia of unknown origin (PUO)
4. Tumor necrosis factor (TNF)
5. Increased production of prostaglandins particularly in hypothalamus. Prostaglandins cause more heat production and loss of heat.

Treatment

1. Use antibiotics in cases of infectious diseases, preferably long-acting antibiotics, such as Terramycin LA, Enromycin LA, etc.
2. Administer anti-inflammatory drugs like Melonex, Flunixin meglumine (unixin of hexter), ketoprofen inj. 100 mg/ml (10–15 ml IV/IM in large animals).
3. Cephalexin with serratopeptidase is better in pus forming infections, such as endometritis, metritis, pyometra, anoestrus and repeat breeding. If there is fever in goats, try Tiamulin first orally or injection for 3 days or erythromycin injection for 3 days, if the fever drops it is a favourable indication of response against mycoplasma (contagious caprine pleuropneumonia or CCPP), example avitia 80% (product of Brihans pharma).

◼ REDUCTION OF CALF MORTALITY TO LESS THAN 20% BY GLOBULIN INJECTIONS

In India, mortality up to 50% has been recorded in large dairy herds. Calf mortality rate of 20% can reduce net profit by 38% (Banerjee GC, *Textbook of Animal Husbandry*, 8th reprint, 2015, p 715). The causes of mortality in order of importance are pneumonia, enteritis, septicaemia/toxaemia, worm infestation, and bloat.

In USA, mortality rate of 6% excluding weak born and stillborn calves is considered best although mortality varies from 2 to 60%. A study conducted in 2002 in USA by National Animal Health Monitoring System found that over 40% of dairy heifer calves had failure of transfer of colostral immunoglobulins. (National Dairy Evaluation Project, Fort Collins, CO, USDA APHIS: VS, 2002).

In India, the average mortality in cow calves below one month was 51.8% (Radhakrishnan KV, 2007, Indian Veterinary Journal, 84, 537–539). Out of these, 21.5% died due to septicaemia.

Any delay beyond the first few hours of life (birth) particularly after 8 hours significantly reduces the amount of immunoglobulin absorbed. The recommendation is that all neonates be fed colostrums within two hours of life. 25 to 34% of calves failed to suck colostrum by 6 to 8 hours of age and 18% did not suck by 18 hours of age. Even after absorption, the half-life of IgG, IgM and IgA are 20, 4, and 2 days respectively, making them vulnerable to disease by 21 days. Protection does not reach to maximum levels until 2 to 3 months age in calves.

Cross Species Colostrum

Bovine colostrum can be fed (injected) to a number of different species. Bovine colostrums has been successfully used for many years to improve survival rate of hysterectomy produced artificially reared pigs. It has also been used as an alternative source of colostral antibodies for rearing goats free from caprine arthritis and encephalitis. Bovine colostrums can provide some protection to newborn foals against neonatal infections.

■ NORMAL TEMPERATURE OF ANIMALS

Species	°C	°F
Cattle up to 1 year	38.5–40.0	101.3–104.0
Cattle above 1 year	37.5–39.5	99.5–101.5
Buffalo	37.5–39.6	99.5–102.2
Camel	35.5–38.6	95.0–101.5
Sheep above 1 year	38.5–40.0	101.3–104.0
Goat (adult)	38.5–40.5	101.3–104.0
Goat (kid)	38.5–41.0	101.3–105.8
Pig (adult)	38.0–40.0	100.4–104.0
dog	37.5–39.0	99.5–102.0
cat	38.0–39.5	100.4–103.1
Poultry (domestic)	40.5–43.0	104.9–109.4
Pigeon	41.0–44.1	105.8–111.4
Horse (adult)	37.5–38.5	99.5–100.4

Fever

- Mild: 1 to 1.5°F above normal
- Moderate: 2.5 to 3°F above normal
- High: 3 to 5°F above normal
- Hyperthermia: 6°F or more above normal.

Old animals may have 1°F temperature below normal. Similarly females have slightly more temperature than males. In late stages of pregnancy the temperature goes up but in bitches it drops by 2–4°F just before delivery.

■ TREATMENT OF PUS FORMING (PYOGENIC) INFECTIONS

Infections resulting in pus formation may occur in wide variety of diseases. Important conditions are pyometra, naval ill (pus in umbbelicus of newborn calf), mastitis, open wound, fractures, etc. in such cases it is dependent on discretion of practitioner to use antibiotics mainly against gram-positive cocci, etc. For example, Dicrysticin-S or Dicrysticin DS (double strength). For Dicrysticin-S add 7.5 ml distilled water in a vial to make 10 ml suspension. This injection covers gram-negative organisms also due to streptomycin. This is economical also. Dose is 2 ml for 50 kg body weight (BW) and 1 ml for 5 kg BW in small animals (Zydus product).

Penicillin G procaine in oil is a long-acting procain penicillin G with aluminium-monistearate for chronic cases or cases requiring long-healing time, such as mastitis, metritis, cystitis, chronic wounds, complicated fractures. (presentation 10 ml having 3,00,000 units; dose is 8000 IU per kg BW. Give deep IM injection with 14 guage needle due to thick suspension). Chloramphenicol can also be given as deep IM injection at the rate of 8–12 mg/kg BW in large animals and 10–15 mg/kg BW for localised pyoderma, pustular dermatitis, foot rot, hoof infection, castration, and yoke galls.

Homoeopathic Medicines for Pus Forming Infections

Hepar sulph 6: In chronic abscesses, recurrent, I treated a case in a man not responding to any treatment even in medical college (multiple recurrent abscesses). Repeated hepar sulph 6 in globules cured the disease.

Hepar sulph 200: 2–4 drops, repeated everyday, if needed; to be given with little water in a clean mouth (1/2 teaspoonful in adult cow, etc).

Silica: Silica alternated with hepar sulph is very good for chronic deep seated purulent infections such as in bone, fistula or mastitis. Mastitis with thick purulent exudates have responded with recovery by repeated doses of Hepar Sulph 200 and silica 200 given alternately by mouth for a few days. This removes clotted purulent exudate.

Initial pus forming lesions: If Hepar Sulph 200 is taken as 3–4 drops in clean mouth it will abort (stop) pimples, abscesses, etc. generally occurring on face or skin of human beings.

Purulent infection in eyes: If there is purulent conjunctivitis give Argentums Nitricum 1000 as 3 to 4 drops by mouth in clean mouth. Nothing should be eaten or tea, coffee should be avoided for at least half- to one-hour before and after taking these medicines.

Dental Infections

Prolonged purulent gingivitis or periodontitis can be cured by repeated doses of Calendula 30 in globules (1 to 2 drops). Dental root infection (deep odontitis) particularly in teeth of lower jaw respond wonderfully to Hekla lava 200, a homoeopathic medicine, taken as few drops have cured pain in my molar (root) giving it a life of 20 years after being shaken (spoiled) by a dentist.

Staphysagria 30 given in repeated doses for a few weeks can even help in regeneration of teeth (particularly molar). Also in case of wisdom tooth.

Septic Metritis

Septic metritis generally develops within 2 to 10 days after parturition in cows. There is fever and fowl smelling purulent discharge. Mixed bacterial infection is generally responsible for the disease. Dystocia and retained placenta predispose to infection as also suppressed immunity or impaired neutrophil function. Retained placenta and septic metritis may not be easily diagnosed. There may be tenesmus, loss of appetite, tachycardia (100 or more heart rate) and toxemia.

Causal bacteria: E coli, Proteus sp, Staphylococcus sp.

Treatment

Intramuscular procaine penicillin: 22000 units per kg BW for 4–5 days or oxytetracyclin injections IV at rate of 11 to 25 mg BW daily. In chronic cases Silica 200, half teaspoonful may be given in water. (PRIN LA injection (Brihans) in 1 gram)

Intrauterine boluses or tablets (they act for 72 hours)

C flox TZ intrauterine (of Intas) or Neovet may be given or Ropitas (Intas) 4 boli may be put into the uterus for releases of placenta in 30 minutes:

1. *URTIS bolus (Van vet):* It is used to treat metritis, endometritis, cervicitis, vaginitis and pyometra and ROP. One or two boli are fed orally twice daily.

2. *Metricare IU:* Contains iodine and metronidazole for indications given for urtis bolus; 30 to 60 ml of this liquid is introduced by IU route and repeated at 24 hours for 2 days (available as bottle 30 and 100 ml).

3. *Oriprim U bolus (Zydus product):* It contains trimethoprim and sulphamethoxazole. Two to four boli are introduced into uterus after parturition. If cervix is not fully open grind and dissolve boli in 30 ml sterile water and infuse into uterus.

'Cleanex' (Dosch, Merial Animal Health, Mumbai)

Cleanex contains nitrofurazone, metronidazole, urea, povidone iodine and nitrofurazone. It is widely effective antibacterial against both aerobic and anaerobic organisms by preventing aerobic and anaerobic metabolism of bacteria. Metronidazole is effective against anaerobic bacteria. Urea dissolves the matrix of reproductive corneal epithelium and thus exposes the hidden bacteria. Povidone iodine denatures bacterial cell proteins and kills the bacteria.

- *Indications:* Endometritis, metritis, pyometra, and retention of placenta.
- *Dose and administration:* 2–4 bolus intrauterine daily for 3 to 5 days.
- *Sheep and goats:* 1 bolus for 3 to 5 days
- *Lenovo AP:* (Product of Neovet/Intas).

Contains levofloxacin, ornidazole, and alphatocopherol in 30 and 60 ml bottles. Indications are repeat breeding, endometritis, metritis, and pyometra (after draining out pus). Introduce 30 ml solution by IU route with the help of full-length hand glove.

▨ NEWBORN OF OTHER SPECIES

Pigs: Somewhat similar steps as suggested for calves may be followed. For hypothermic newborn piglets a warm box heated by electric lamps will be good along with intraperitoneal injection of glucose and tonophosphan, etc. box having warmth of 33 to 37°C for three days will provide better results.

Sheep: Sheep are more prone to exposure to *heat and humidity* because of insulation provided by wool, humidity of 34 to 40 mm Hg can be fatal. It is therefore essential to provide cold water, shade and tranquilisers (Phytocool of Natural Remedies), increased doses of vitamin C, homoeopathic medicine 'Glonoine 30' may be mixed in cold drinking water at the rate of 2 teaspoonful per 50 sheeps or we use a mixture of 4 homoeopathic medicines in equal quantity is given below:

- Glonoine 6
- Selenium 6
- Coca 6
- Naja 30

Two teaspoonfuls of this mixture are to be given in drinking water for 50 cows or 100 goats or sheep. In the evening we administer Dualcamara 200 in same dose rate (two teaspoonfuls) in drinking water.

Another allopathic combination named "Replina" of TTK (animal welfare division, 39, oliver road mylapore, Chennai 600004, India) was used in June 2017 at the rate of 1 g in 2 litre water for cattle and was found to be moderately effective. This mixture is initially produced for use in poultry and for use in large animals the manufactures may be consulted. Contents of replina are sodium salicylate, glycine and protein hydrolysate, sodium bicarbonate, sodium citrate, magnesium chloride, sodium potassium chloride, calcium lactate and vitamin C.

PYREXIA (FEVER) OF UNKNOWN ORIGIN

Pyrexia of unknown origin (PUO) as it is called is rather common in cow calves and buffalo calves. Fever or PUO is pyrexia due to undiagnosed cause.

Usual undetected causes are:
1. Theleriasis (in our experiences)
2. Pyogenic infections such as metritis, pericarditis, pyelonephritis, pleurisy, etc.

Treatment

In my experiences here at Surat Panjarapole which has a population of around 5000 to 6000 old or male calves, etc. I use injections of:
1. Oxytetracycline long-acting (Zydus) at the rate of 1 ml per kg BW
2. Barenil (MSD product).

Barenil covers babesiosis, trypanosomiasis and theleriosis. These two injections are given simultaneously, Barenil is given at the dose rate of 5 to 10 ml per 100 kg BW. Other antiprotozoal injections are Zubion (intas), prozomin (Virbac product), Trityl (Lyca product), Nilbery and Zokil (Mankind). Zokil is also used at dose rate of Barenil.

If pyogenic infections are suspected in the body than I prefer "Metra" a herbal product of Tineta Pharma, which is, an oral preparation (500 ml and 1 lit). The dose is 75 to 100 ml daily for a large animal and 50 ml per day for a small animal. It prevents infection, expels remains of placenta, etc. and reduces inflammation.

Another approach with homoeopathic medicine is to give antibiotics of long-acting type like terramycin or enromycin (like "fortivir" of virbac, "Kenro 120" of Kepler which acts for 96 hours, Vetazo (ceftriaxone + tazobactem) of Zydus acts both on gram-positive and gram-negative organisms (2250 mg: or 3375 mg vials) dose 5–10 mg per kg by IM or IV route, dose in sheep and goats is 250 to 300 mg, 'Vetdox Forte' of Zydus is also good for gram-positive and gram-negative bacteria and is very good for septicaemia and pneumonia. Dissolve 2 g vial content in 10 ml distilled water, inject IM or IV (300 mg in sheep and goats or 5 to 10 mg/kg body weight in other animals). Give injections for 3 to 5 days.

Dicrysticin-and Dicrysticin-DS

It contains streptomycin sulphate 5 g and procaine penicillin G 35,00,000 units and penicillin G sodium 100,00,000 units. It is a reputed drug being used for decades against ailments caused by gram-positive and gram-negative infections such as listed below:
1. Fever
2. Septicaemia
3. Arthritis

4. Pneumonia   5. Naval illness   6. Diarrhoea
7. Dysentery   8. Conjunctivitis, etc.

Veterinarian's first choice in mixed infections (supreme synergy of penicillin and streptomycin)

Composition: Each vial of Dicrysticin-s contains
- Streptomycin sulphate   2.5 g of base
- Procaine penicillin G   15,00,000 units
- Penicillin G sodium   500,000 units

Indication: Dicrysticin is highly effective against a wide variety of gram-positive and gram-negative bacteria as well as mixed infections (infections of unknown origin).

Cattle and calf: Pneumonia, foot rot, peritonitis, abscesses, uterine infections, urinary tract infections, postcastration infections, infectious calf scours, complications of mastitis and bacillary dysentery.

Pig: Infectious scours, bloody diarrhoea, naval infection, postcastration infections, wound infections, erysipelas.

Sheep and goat: Infectious scours, pneumonia, naval infections, castration and docking infections, complications of mastitis and wound infections.

Horse: Strangles, infectious scours, naval infections, castration and wound infections, abscesses, pneumonia, urinary tract infections.

Dog: Infectious diarrhoea, otitis externa, pneumonia, secondary bacterial infections.

Preparation: Add 7.5 ml of sterile distilled water to each vial of dicrysticin-s to make 10 ml suspension.

Add 15 ml of sterile distilled water to each vial of dicrysticin –DS to make 20 ml suspension.

Dosage and administration: Large animals 2 ml/50 kg BW (IM)
Small animals 1 ml/5 kg BW (IM).

Penicillin G procaine in oil (PAM injection) penetrating attack on microorganisms for prolonged action.

Long-acting sterile procaine penicillin G with Aluminium Monostearate (96 hours).

Composition: Each ml contains
- Procaine Penicillin G USP 3,00,000 unitts
- Aluminium Monostearate USP 2%.

Action and Absorption: Because of its low water solubility, procaine penicillin G is slowly absorbed by the tissues absorption takes place more slowly but more uniformly. Procaine penicillin G in oil produces persistent penicillin levels in blood. A significant level in blood along with action is maintained up to 96 hours after administration. The absorption of procaine penicillin G in oil may be delayed but its effect is due to delayed excretion.

Indications

Treatment of conditions caused by organisms with low penicillin resistance, particularly that requiring prolonged drug exposure like mastitis, metritis, cystitis, abscesses, chronic wounds and skin infections, postcastration infections, anthrax, haemorrhagic septicaemia, black quarter, strangles and naval ill.

Dosage and administration: Panicillin or Dicrysticine (40,000 IU per Kg BW) is better for good results.

Large and medium sized animals: 8000 IU/kg BW.

Enz. Pneumonia: Penicillin G procaine in oil injection (Zydus product). It acts for 96 hours per injection.

Dogs and cats: 300000–600000 IU per animal for at least 3 days to be administered by deep IM only. Change the site for each injection. Use 14 gauge needles for cattle and horses, 18 gauge for sheep, goat, pig and 20 gauge for dogs and cats. The needle and syringe should be thouroughly sterilized by boiling in water before use or use disposable sterile syringe and needle.

Shake the vial well to ensure uniform suspension. Inject air into the vial for easier withdrawal. Do not massage the site of injection. Not more than 10 ml should be injected at one site.

Indications: Mastitis, metritis, cystitis, abscesses, chronic wounds, postcastration, anthrax, HS, BQ naval illness.

Vetclox forte (hard on infections, soft on pocket) broad-spectrum combination of ampicillin and cloxacillin.

Composition: Each ml contains
- Ampicillin sodium IP (equivalent to anhydrous ampicillin) 1 g
- Cloxacillin sodium IP (equivalent to anhydrous cloxacillin) 1 g.

Antibacterial Spectrum

Wide spectrum of action over gram-positive and gram-negative bacteria, including beta lactamase producing bacteria which are decisively eliminated. Cloxacillin, a penicillin derivative, acts against gram-positive bacteria and also lends support to ampicillin activity. It is also active against Clostridia, Salmonella, Shigella, and *E. coli.* besides the pyogenic infections mentioned above.

Indications: Cattle, sheep and goat.

Pneumonia, septicaemia, enteritis, colitis, coliform and other types of bacterial mastitis, urogenital infections, foot wounds, dermatitis.

Horse: Enteritis in foals, urinary tract infections, respiratory infections and post surgical wounds.

Dogs and cats: Enteritis, dermatitis, ear infections, respiratory tract infections, post surgical infections and urogenital infections.

Dosage and administration: Add 10 ml of distilled water to make the solution. recommended dose is 5–10 mg/kg BW. Repeat after 24 hours for 3–5 days. Administered by IM or IV route.

Steclin Injection (Zydus product): Ready to use solution of oxytetracyclin 50 mg per ml.

Acts against gram-positive and gram-negative organisms.

Calf, cattle, buffalo: Abscesses, actinomycosis, actinobacillosis, anthrax, BQ calf diarrhoea, enteritis, foot-lot, metritis, urogenital infections, complications of viral disease.

Horses: As above plus dental infections, strangles, pneumonia.

Pig: Almost all infectious diseases including leptospirosis.

Sheep and goats: As for cattle, buffaloes, plus leptospirosis, ear infections, pneumonia.

Dosage

- Large animals: 5–10 mg/kg BW (1–2 ml/25 kg).
- Small animals: 7–11 mg/kg BW.
- Route: IM, IV, SC.

■ CALF SCOURS (DIARRHOEA) AND DYSENTERY

Diarrhoea of newborn calves is the most common disease and may affect up to 75% in intensive dairy farming or in poorly managed dairy establishments. In average kind of dairy farm 30% of newborn calves may be affected with mortality varying from 10–50% but usually around 25%. The calves should be dewormed regularly every month for a period of 6 months.

Pigs: About 6%, more likely before weaning.

Kids: Born underweight or colostrums deprived.

Major Causes of Diarrhoea

Bacteria: Escherichia coli
             Salmonella pullorum
             Salmonella typhimurium
             Salmonella enteritidis
             Proteus vulgaris
             Staphylococcus spp.
             Streptococcus spp.
             Clostridium perfringens

Consequences of Diarrhoea: Loose and frequent defecation, sometimes containing mucus and/or blood; increased water loss, resulting in dehydration; loss of electrolytes; decreased abomasal pH (acidosis) and; disturbed intestinal flora and loss of integrity of intestinal mucous membrane.

Parasites: Nematodes like Ascaris suum and Oestertagia oestertagi

Protozoa: Eimeria bovis and other Eimeria spp Cryptosporidium spp.

Virus: Rota virus, Corona virus.

Causes and risk factors
1. Calves up to 3 days age.
2. Feeding colostrums (warm) preferably as early as 6–12 hours after birth, twice a day.
3. More than 80% cases of diarrhoea are caused by K99 entertoxic *E. coli*, usually before 4 days of birth.
4. Calves born to heifers are 4 times at risk than those born to cows.
5. Calf must drink 80 to 100 ml colostrums and better 150 ml colostrums within a few hours after birth but the quantity of immunoglobulins differ from 2 to 150 g per litre depending on breed (average is 40 to 50 mg per ml). High milk producers like Holstein fresian have less globulins in colostrums. Hence, it is advisable to give injections of globulins in valuable calves. Inject 8 to 10 g

immunoglobulins subcutaneously in such calves, as shown in the research paper presented by the first author. The Veterinary Communications, July 2010 and Indian Association of Veterinary Pathologists Annual Conference, date 11-11-2016, selected for P.P. Gupta Award.

6. Some cows specially of imported breeds may ignore the newborn calf, regarding feeding of colostrums.

7. Mixed infection: It generally occurs at around 1 to 2 week age affecting about 50% calves. Mixed infection is due to *E. coli*, cryptosporidium and corona virus. There is fluid diarrhoea and death due to dehydration.

8. Change of diet (milk replacer) and overfeeding with milk.

9. Rotaviral diarrhoea: Bovine rotavirus (type A to G, 7 types) may affect 30 to 40% neonatal calves within 2 weeks after birth. Type A infection is most common and type B and G in India. Faeces may be semi liquid or liquid. The source of infection is adult or calves.

10. Coronaviral diarrhoea: This infection mostly occurs at 1 to 2 weeks age, more in winter. The source of virus are carrier cows. The virus has only one serotype.

11. Diarrhoea of unknown origin: Sometimes the cause of diarrhoea may not be discovered. In such cases two treatments may succeed:

    i. Biochemic mixture of medicines given on page 19.

    ii. Rocklow bolus (Kepler Vet Mission Pvt Ltd) for diarrhoea and dysentery of unknown origin 1 bolus/100 kg BW for 3 to 5 days (contains ofloxacin 1000 mg + Ornidazole 1800 mg).

    Floratone Bolus (Concept product): It is available as 6 bolus strip. It is antidiarrhoeas medicine—diarrhoea may be due to indigestion acidosis, destruction of microflora of rumen. Dose for calf, sheep, and goat is 1/2 to 1 bolus per calf, sheep or goat for 3–5 days.

    iii. Cobactan 2.5% injection, a 4th generation cephalosporin injection is good (for calf septicaemia 2 ml/25 kg BW IM daily for 3–5 days. Other bacterial infection: 1 ml/25 kg BW IM daily for 2–5 days).

    Nonspecific treatment: KOL and KOL-L (Carus Labs Pvt Ltd) are good.

Differential Diagnosis

Agent	Age of disease	Type of diarrhoea	Season	Faeces	Sporadic	Outbreak	Mortality
E. coli	Within 4 to 7 days	Foul smell with liquid or pasty or undigested milk	Any season	Semiliquid	Yes	No	High
Rota virus	Within 7days to 2 weeks	Liquid or pasty	Any season	Semiliquid or pasty	No	Outbreak	9–60%
Corona virus Bovine viral diarrhoea BVD	3 to 6 weeks	Liquid or pasty	Winter (more)	Semiliquid or pasty	No	Yes + Rinderpest like erosions in mouth	50 to 100% (imp)

Histopathologically there is atrophy of both small and large intestinal epithelium from columnar to cuboidal or flat (squamous).

Treatment

Due to use of injections of colostral immunoglobulins we have rarely if ever treated cases of diarrhea where there is population of 11000 to 12000 cattle kept at Tharoli and Akhakhole branches of Shri Surat Panjrapole, Surat. Diarrhoea but occurs often in sheep and goats.

Drugs used to treat diarrhoea

Vetfur-TL (Dosch, Merial Animal Health): Contains Metrinidazole, furazolidone and leperomide hydrochloride. Metronidazole kills anaerobic, mainly clostridial organisms. Furazolidine is effective against both aerobic and anaerobic organisms. Leperomide affects myentric plaxus of intestine like morphine which reduces mobility of intestine responsible for expulsion of fecal matter and allows time for intestine to absorb water (prevent dehydration).

Indications

1. Diarrhoea of bacterial origin
2. Protozoal infections (metronidazole)
3. Inflammatory bowel disease.
   It comes in packaging 10 × 4 bolus
   Large animal: 4–6 bolus for 3–5 days
   Small animal: 1–2 bolus for 3–5 days

Cflox-TZ (Intas): Contains ciprofloxacin and tinidazole which cover wide range of bacterial and protozoal diarrhoea. Available as strips of 10 tablets or box of 25 strips. It is also effective against enterotoxaemia (not the toxins), Salmonella and partly in JD. It treats Giardial, Proteus and Pseudomonas infections also.

Dose: Sheep, goats, calves—
1. Tablet per 15–25 kg BW for 3–5 days.
2. Tablets for 30–40 kg BW for 3–5 days.

Sheep, goat and calves

Griptol-N (Intas): Contains levofloxacin and ornidazole (60 ml bottle) which is effective against bacterial, protozoal diarrhoea (aerobic and anaerobic) including amoeba, coccidia (Eimeria, etc.), particularly in pets.

Dose: 1 ml/4 kg body weight
6 ml/25 kg body weight (sheep, goats)

Care Bolus (Vet Care product—antibacterial, antifungal, and antiprotozoal): Effective against *E. coli*, Salmonella, Staphylococci, Streptococci, Entamoeba, *Eimeria coccidia*.

Dose: ½ to 1 bolus per calf, sheep, goat, in cases of diarrhoea, dysentery; aerobic and anaerobic infections.

Floratone bolus: Antidiarrhoeal medicine against indigestion, acidosis, rumen microflora destruction. Calf, sheep, goat—1/2 to 1 bolus TDS; 3–5 times daily. Comes in 6 boli strip.

BVD bolus (Ceva Polchem Pvt Ltd): It is best product which multipurpose (mixed bacterial infections, dysentery, coccidiosis, Giardiasis, Salmonellosis, Trichamonas abortion and Amoebiasis. Dose 1 bolus per 50 kg BW orally for 3–5 days.

Other drugs are Lycip, Heloquinol (Vet Care), Lyphovet (Lyka), Lyfovet (injection)

1. Prevention both against bacterial and viral diarrhoea is feeding, clean, warm colostrums soon after birth.
2. Treatment of any type of diarrhoea by a combination of 9 type of biochemical medicine by me has been found to be most successful in any type of diarrhoea. The mixture called "cholera mixture" is used for the treatment of cholera-like symptoms in man. It consists of a mixture of the following biochemical tablets in equal proportion (number). These are available from any homoeopathic medicine shop and very cheap. These tablets should be finely powdered and kept in dry container or bottle almost indefinitely. This mixture stops diarrhoea in any species including humans within minutes to half an hour. I have invariably cured my own diarrhoea and of friends for the last 40 years of my practice in homoeopathy.
   a. Kalimur 3X
   b. Natrum phos 3X
   c. Kali phos 3X
   d. Magnesia phos 3X
   e. Calcaria phos 3X
   f. Natrum mur 3X
   g. Ferrum phos 3X
   h. Kali sulph 3X
   (equal parts/number of tablets of each)
   The finely ground powder may be dissolved preferably in hot (not boiling) water for better and quick action. Take about a good pinch of the powder (about 2 g). In urgency, the powder may even be put on the tongue and allowed to dissolve slowly in mouth. In animals half teaspoonful of biochemic powder dissolved in water may be given by mouth, at half hour interval or 1 hourly or 3 times a day depending on severity of diarrhoea. If fever is also recorded, antibiotic injections like dicrysticin can be given. As a control measure, some powder may be mixed in drinking water of healthy and sick animals.
3. *Clampivet-D* (ampicillin dicloxacillin injection) can be given at the rate of 4–10 mg/kg BW twice daily by IV or IM and repeated after 6 to 8 hours.
   Floserm (levofloxacin) injection can also be used. See other drugs in the important list of medicines.

Chapter 3

Important Infectious Diseases

■ BOVINE VIRAL DIARRHOEA (BVD)/ MUCOSAL DISEASE/ PESTIVIRUS DISEASE

Cause: Bovine Viral Diarrhoea Virus (BVDV)

BVD affects 3 to 6 weeks old calves (more age than the hosts described for diarrhoea above).

Symptoms

- Usually mild or symptomless
- Affects 6–24 month old cattle
- Sometimes (rarely) fever, erosions in mouth, abomasum.

Clinical Pathology

- Leucopenia (in acute form)
- Thrombocytopenia (causing widespread haemorrhages)
- *Morbidity:* 25% or less
- *Mortality:* 80% of sick calves (low morbidity high mortality).

■ SUPPORTIVE TREATMENT FOR DIARRHOEA

1. ORS or ORT calf powder (Carus lab pvt ltd) should be given along with curative treatment given above to prevent dehydration if needed.
2. Intraperitoneal method may be adopted in case of seriously sick calves.
3. Ayurvedic and homoeopathic drugs such as given below may be used along with cholera mixture if needed but these medicines may be given at least 1 hour after or before biochemic mixture.
   a. Croton 6 or 30: A homoeopathic medicine acts very well and compliments the "cholera mixture". This is given in 3–4 drops in mouth or in sugar globules.
   b. Jondilla (a homoeopathic combination in syrup form; product of Medisynth company). Restorative in gastric and hepatic complaints. It improves appetite and digestion. I give 1 teaspoonful before milk or milk replacer feeding.

■ DYSENTERY

Dysentery means passing of liquid or semiliquid faeces with mucous fibrin and or blood. Such infections occur as listed below:
- *Calves:* Due to *E. coli*, milk of mastitis affected cow
- *Sheep and goats:* Coccidiosis
- *Adult cattle:* Salmonellosis (bad odour)
- *Haemorrhagic enteritis:* PPR, pasteurellosis, enterotoxaemia in sheep and goats.

Animals make grunting sound due to pain and faeces is passed out with straining.

Diagnosis

1. Presence of blood, mucous or fibrin in faeces.
2. Fecal examination to detect causal bacteria or coccidial schizonts (cysts are seen in chronic case).
3. Large number of *Clostridium perfringens* by methylene blue or gram's staining of fecal smears (in enterotoxemia of sheep, goats, calves (type b and c of *Clostridium Perfringens*), piglets (necrotic enteritis) and foals. Organisms are so many that they look like smear from pure culture.

Treatment

1. Colostrums feeding (as preventive) from vaccinated mother.
2. Oral doses of penicillin G or amoxicillin along with injections of dicrysticine.
3. Mixture of 9 types of biochemic medicines as described above + Croton 6 drops (homoeopathic).
4. *Cipro –TZ tablets* are very good in my experience.

Homoeopathic and Biochemic Treatment

1. The drug of choice in bloody dysentery is mercury corrosivus (Mercor) 200. It is given as 3–5 drops in calves sheep and goats and ½ teaspoonful in adult cattle, twice a day.
2. Aloe 200 works better in milder cases without blood, dose and other methods are as for merc or 200.
3. *Dysentery mixture no 9 (Biochemic):* Given as directed by manufracturer. Generally 4–6 tablets 3 times in a day in water or honey.
4. *Griptol – N:* Contains levofloxacin + ornidazole. It is basically meant for dogs but I have found it good along with cholera powder (given in clean mouth and not mixed with Griptol) for treatment of diarrhoea in sheep and goats and young calves. It is given at the rate of 1 ml per 4 kg body weight, morning, evening for 3 to 5 days.
5. *C flox TZ (Intas product):* It covers wide range of gastrointestinal pathogens. They are available as boli and tablets, powder and injections. It is good for all types of bacterial diarrhoea (salmonella, Johns' diseases, enteritis, giardial infection, Proteus, Pseudomonas infections, CCPP, etc.)
   C flox powder: 15 ml/300 kg BW for 3–5 days by IM or IV route.
   C flox TZ bolus: 1 bolus/300 kg/3–5 days/orally.
   C flox TZ tablets: 1 tablet for sheep, goat, calf/3–5 days orally.
   C flox TZ IU: 60 ml by intrauterine route for pyometra, metritis, ROP, prolapse of uterus.
6. *3 care bolus (Vetcare product):* It contains heloquinol, best advantage is that it is antibacterial, antifungal and antiprotozoal (coccidian, giardia, amoeba)
   Dose: ½ calf bolus/twice daily/3–5 days (strip of 6 bolus).
7. *Floratone bolus (Concept product):* Contains ingredients for simple indigestion, change of food, too much greens, etc. (contains sodium bicarbonate, mag trisilicate, methionine, dextrose, yeast, cobalt, copper, nicotinamide, yeast, sodium phosphate). Packing 4 boli per strip, Dose: calf, sheep, goat 1 bolus/day, cattle: 4 boli/day.
8. *Lykacetin injection (Lyka):* It is a broad-spectrum chloramphenicol injection which has low bacterial resistance.

3G vial: Dose 2–4 mg/kg BW/IV or 20–30 mg/kg/IM inj.
9. *Effigest bolus* (Hester product) similar to floratone bolus
Dose: As for Floratone presentation: Strip of 10

▋ BLACK QUARTER (Black Leg)

This is a world wide disease but of little significance (in my view).

Cause

Clostridium chauvoei, a gram-positive spore forming organism. It survives for several years in soil due to resistant spores. It is more common in rainy season.

Hosts

Cattle of 6 months to 2 years age (young) and sheep more affected after wound infection or without wound. Vaccine is available in India in all states.

Symptoms and Pathology

There is lameness and swelling of upper part of hindlimb or forelimb. Death occurs in 100% cases. The muscles have crepitating swelling due to formation of gas and coffee coloured, fowl smelling fluid. Affected muscles become black (black leg). Death is due to bacterial toxins.

Treatment

Penicillin or dicrysticin is good in high dose (40,000 IU per kg BW) to protect animals in the herd 10,000 IU of penicillin may be injected along with vaccination. Antiserum if available may also be injected subcutaneously in animals in contact.

▋ ANTHRAX

Anthrax is a global disease but in India it is rarely observed, possibly due to available vaccine. Sixty per cent cases were reported from developing countries in 2004.

Cause

Bacillus anthracis it has a glutamic capsule which stops phagocytosis. It also produces oedema factor (fector I) lethal/killer factor II and a antigenic/protective factor III. Tropical countries like India and south Asia have more chances of disease.

Hosts

Cattle (important) sheep, pigs and horses. Localised as swellings and intestinal inflammation. Humans can also be infected by cuts or inhalation of infective dust, wool, etc.

Infection

By mouth from soil having anthrax spores, or by inhalation and rarely by biting insects. Climatic changes, such as start of rain, calcium rich soils and stagnant water help infections.

Symptoms

One has to be extremely careful when diagnosing anthrax because it occurs in 2 forms.

Per acute form: Usually as an outbreak, the animals may die without showing signs, within 1–2 hours. Fever due to septicaemia is often seen (up to 107° F) with convulsions, dyspnoea and sounds of agony. One very often and significant sign is bleeding from nostrils, anus, vulva or mouth.

I came across a case of per acute form in Ranchi in 1990 which a person brought his dead cow with bleeding from all natural orifices. A teenaged boy also came along who looked shocked. The owner told that the cow had been crying and struggling with the rope of its neck partly entangled and the owner came out of the house and found the boy trying to pacify the cow in agony. Soon after the cow died hence the owner thought that the boy had poisoned the animal resulting in the death of the cow. The owner took the child to a police station and had filed an FIR against the child who was shocked and too spellbound to argue.

The owner of the cow requested me to examine and give openion on the cause of death so the child may be protected or prosecuted. I concluded that:

a. The cow had died due to peracute anthrax as shown by bleeding from nostrils, mouth and vagina.

b. Presence of bacilli in the oozed out blood.

c. Sudden death within a few minutes.

The boy's role in the supposed poisioning was ruled out because there is no poison which could have killed the cow within the few minutes he was near the cow. Secondly, the boy had no reason to poison the cow (being an unknown stranger). The owner withdrew the FIR and the boy was happy to get relief from an unexpected harassment.

Prevention and Treatment

Vaccination: Vaccination is the cheapest and reliable for control/prevention of anthrax.

1. *Anthrax spore vaccine* (available from Institute of Biological Product, Veterinary college, MHOW, Indore, MP) is injected in the dose of 1 ml subcut in growing and adult cattle, sheep and goats.

2. *After infection:* The carcass should not be opened, only a smear from blood exudate or from ear vein should be stained with polychrome methylene blue which shows stout bacilli with light blue coloured capsule. Organisms form short chains (Fig. 3.1).

Anthrax in human beings: Anthrax can also produce serious infection in man as respiratory disease (wool sorters disease) or as an acute subcutaneous infection, mostly in farmers, veterinarians, etc. In skin, the leision is called malignant carbuncle.

Treatment: Oxytetracyclin 5 mg/kg BW SC/or IM; other drugs are ampicillin and azithromycin.

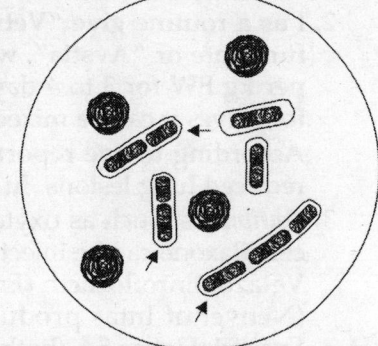

Fig. 3.1: Capsulated anthrax bacilli (arrow) in blood

3. In much putrified carcass a piece of skin may be taken to prepare a fine trichurate in normal saline to act as antigen for ASCOLI's precipitation test.

Disposal of Carcass

Anthrax affected carcass should be handled carefully since it can produce disease in humans also. Carcass, blood and soil of the areas should be collected and buried in at least 2 meter deep trench and covered with quicklime. The place of sickness of animal should be disinfected by heat (above 60° C) by burning straw or dry leaves for few minutes. On the floor 5% Lysol or 5 % formalin should be spread out as soon after death of the animal as possible. Since anthrax bacteria sporulate in a few hours which remain alive for decades. Clothes, wool, etc. should be sterilised by dipping in 10 % formaldehyde for 18 to 20 hours.

Treatment

Sick animal may not recover inspite of treatment, unless suspected in very early stage. Penicillin (procaine penicillin G and sodium penicillin 15,000 IU and 5,00,000 IU respectively) should be injected IM at every 24 hours (4000 IU per kg body weight). FPP 20 and FPP 40 of Zydus are ideal. Dicrysticin S of Zydus is also good. Inject

DC-DS at the rate of 2 ml per kg body weight. Treat for 5 days to avoid relapse. (FPP = Fortified procaine penicillin; dose: 4000 units/kg body weight at 24 hour interval)

ENZOOTIC PNEUMONIA OF CALVES

Enzootic pneumonia is a febrile disease of lungs due to mixed infections, in dairy calves during nursing or neonatal age.

Etiology

It is a disease due to mixed infection of Mycoplasma species (M. bovis). Parainfluenza virus (PI3) and other respiratory viruses such as bovine respiratory syncytial virus (BRSV).

Symptoms

The disease affects calves under 3–5 months of age. Many calves become sick but mortality is low. This is not very important condition provided warm colostrum is fed within a few hours after birth. I give subcut injections of globulin prepared by me (senior author). Mortality can be as high as 30%, particularly in winter.

Prevention and Treatment

1. Feed fresh colostrum soon after birth.
2. I as a routine give "Vetmulin" (Huvepharma product) 80% tiamulin hydrogen fumarate or "Avstia", which can be given in feed or water at the rate of 50 mg per kg BW for 3 to 4 days after birth or after arrival (in case of sheep and goats, for calves it can be mixed in milk.)
   According to one report 10 mg of tiamutin per kg BW for 10 days significantly reduced lung lesions. In goats higher dose 20 mg/kg BW may be given.
3. *Antibiotics:* Such as oxytetracyclin long acting (LA) and Trimethoprim (oriprime) ceftrilaxone can be injected at the rate of 10 mg/kg BW (IM/II IV), e.g. Zydaceph, Vetazo. Enrofloxacin (Enrodac-10) at the rate of 5 mg per kg BW. Intaceph Tazo (Neovet of Intas product) is very good (10 mg/kg BW/IM or IV for 5 days). Enrogil, Flobac SA (both long-acting) are also good and injected IM/IV/SC at the rate of 30 to 40 ml per 300–400 kg BW. Their range of effectiveness is given below:

Pasteurella	Haemophilus	Mycoplasma	E. coli	Samonella	Klebsiella	Proteus
+++	+++	+++	+++	+++	+++	+++

Homoeopathic Drugs

Homoeopathic drugs are used as complimentary for treatment of pneumonia. I use the following medicines: Phosphorus 200, Bryonia 200, or Balladonna 1000, a few drops per animal in water twice a day.

■ HAEMORRHAGIC SEPTICAEMIA (HS)

It is a well known disease of India and South Asian countries. Less important in USA, Australia, New Zealand.

Mortality

50 to 100% in septicaemic pasteurellosis, more common in rainy season. Bacteria are outside the body. Infection occurs through food, grass, etc. Up to 45% of survivors are carriers (Latent infection).

Hosts

Cattle, buffaloes and pigs.

Symptoms (Fig. 3.2)

- Fever up to 106 to 107° F
- Excessive salivation
- Hot, painful swelling of throat (local name is "Galghotu" disease), neck and brisket
- Dyspnoea (respiratory distress)
- Occasionally bloody diarrhoea (gastroenteritis).

Etiology

Pasteurella Multocida (*P. multocida* asian serotype B: 2,5. These are bipolar gram-negative organisms, typically seen in saliva, fluid of throat swelling and blood smears only in late stage) even by 1% methylene blue staining (Fig. 3.3).

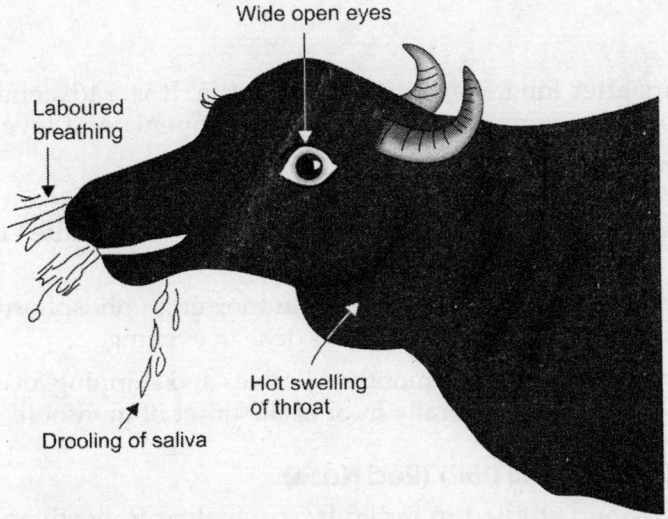

Fig. 3.2: Symptoms of haemorrhagic septicaemia

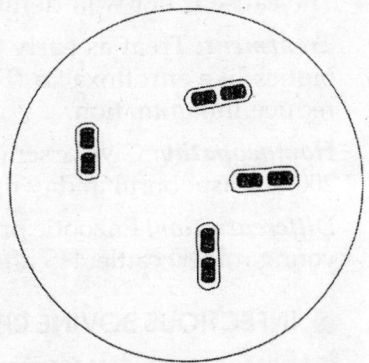

Fig. 3.3: Bipolar pasteurella organisms

Diagnosis

1. *Postmortem:* Haemorrhagic consolidation of lungs, haemorrhagic abomasitis and enteritis, oedema of interstitial tissue of lungs; enlarged haemorrhagic lymph nodes of thorax and throat.
2. Injection of infected blood or throat exudates (0.2 ml) by SC route will kill mice in 24 to 36 hours.
3. Culture of *P. multocida* on laboratory serum enriched culture media from bone marrow because in bone marrow, the organisms survive longest and free from putrefactive bacteria.
4. AGPT and ELISA tests are simple and reliable. (Elisa identifies specific serotypes).

Prevention

Preventive, killed alum precipitated vaccines are available in India, we get our vaccine from Government Institute of Animal Health, Rasalpura, MHOW, Indore MP (Fax 07324-273602), Phone: 07324-273602. It is also available from Institure of Animal Health and Veterinary Biologicals, Hebbal Bangalore 560024.

Vaccine dose is 5 ml, SC injection in adult cattle and buffaloes preferably before onset of rains. Immunity is expected to last for 12 months hence repeated yearly.

Treatment

It is a serious contagious disease requiring immediate treatment of infected and in contact animals in a herd. I had recently treated/controlled an outbreak in a dairy herd with Intaceph Tazo (Intas product) in dose of 5–10 mg/kg BW or Enrofloxacin (Enrocin LA, Enrogyl LA). Enrofloxacin also kills haemophilus, Mycoplasma and Klebsiella. "Enrostrong PZ"(Mankind) is also available as 5 g (single dose) vial. "Flobac,SA" As a single dose (Intas) is sufficient for treatment. Febrifuges like "Meloxicam", "Megludyne" and "Cortalife" may also be injected to stop inflammation. Disinfection of premises: By common disinfectants like formalin 3% or phenyl.

Variants of Respiratory Diseases Similar to *P. Haemolytica* Infections

▨ SHIPPING FEVER

Not common in India. It occurs after long transportation of cattle. It is a toxaemic bronchopneumonia with dyspnoea, cough, leukopenia and neutropenia and fever. The cause is not well-defined.

Treatment: Treat as early as possible. Treat with broad-spectrum long-acting anti-biotics like enrofloxacin (Flobac SA), Enrocin LA with "Megludyne", "contalife" to reduce inflammation.

Homoeopathy: Give arsenicum album 1000, ½ teaspoonful in morning , phosphorus 200 ½ teaspoonful in day time and hepar sulph 200 in same dose in evening.

Differentiation: Enzootic pneumonia affects 2 to 6 month old calves and shipping fever young (older) cattle. HS affects adult cattle, generally in or at the onset of monsoon.

▨ INFECTIOUS BOVINE RHINOTRACHEITIS (IBR) (Red Nose)

It is a common disease observed and studied in india, It is prevalent in north and south India and eastern states.

Etiology

IBR virus bovine herpes virus 1 (BHV1), variants BHV 1-1, BHV1-2.

Hosts

All age groups of cattle, usually as outbreak. In goats, pigs and buffaloes mild disease occurs. The disease exists in wild ruminants as reservoirs.

Mode of Infection

Through grass, feed, and water, semen can transmit infection. Carrier cattle may start infection after, transportation, stress and corticosteroid treatment.

Pathology

Sites of lesions are conjunctiva (pink eye disease), nose, larynx, sometimes meningo-encephalitis (spread from nose). Lungs if affected may result in fatal pneumonia. Affected parts become congested, swollen and there is mucopurulent discharge, mainly from nose, eyes and vagina.

Clinical Signs

Signs may be variable and confusing.

Symptoms

Due to multiple sites of infection the symptoms may be variable but respiratory form is most common.

Respiratory Form

As the name of the disease indicates nasal laryngeal, tracheal inflammation oedema, mucus nasal discharge is seen. Later the nasal discharge becomes mucopurulent. Due to nasal obstruction mouth breathing with protruding tongue may be seen. Inflamed nasal mucosa results in the name " Red nose". Carrier status may exist after recovery. Mortality is low about 1%.

Reproductive Form

In cows vulvovaginitis with redness swelling and formation papules and occasionally abortion.

Treatment: There is no specific treatment. Only three approaches can be taken:
1. Treat with antibiotics to prevent secondary bacterial infections. Recovery is usual after 3 to 5 days.
2. Non-steroid anti inflammatory medicines like "Megludyne" and "contalife" injections.
3. *Homoeopathic:* Give ½ teaspoonful of arsenicum album in drinking water and ½ teaspoonful of phosphorus 200 in small quantity of water twice daily. Keep a gap of at least 30 minutes between the drugs.

Vaccine: There is no vaccine available.

▋ ALLERGIC RHINITIS

This respiratory, nasal and tracheal inflammation ocuurs mostly in autmn when there is flowering of crops or plants. The pollens produce inflammation due to allergy.

Fungus in humid straw may also produce such disease due to allergic response to inhaled fungus.

Symptoms: Sudden dyspnoea, due to formation of mucous and later purulant discharge from nose.

Treatment: Remove the animals away from flowering area or crop area:
1. Antihistaminic injections like Avil and Anistamin (Intas)—both contain chlorpheniramine maleate 10 mg/ml. Inject SC 0.4 to 2 mg/kg BW BD Avilin Vet (MSD) 22.5 mg pheniramine/ml. Inject 5 to 10 ml SC.
2. *Homoeopathy:* Arsenicum album in water as described above and Apis mel 200 in place of phosphorus given as above. Bromium 30, 1/2 teaspoonful in water 2–3 times a day is very good too.
   Other antiallergic drugs are the following:
   • Hisloc 30 and 100 ml (Cadila) injection
   • Cadistin 30 and 100 ml (Zydus) injection
   • Histanil—10, 30, and 100 ml (Vetindia) injection
   • Zeet—30 and 100 ml (Alembic) injection
   • Alert vet—30 and 100 ml (Morvel) injection.

▇ CONTAGIOUS CAPRINE PLEUROPNEUMONIA (CCPP)

1. As soon as new lot of sheep and goats comes to premises they are administered tiamutin (see under enzootic pneumonia). Tiamutin (80%) or Tiamulin I give orally in jaggary in the dose of 250 to 300 mg per adult sheep and goat (about 10 mg per kg BW) for three days to kill mycoplasma in latent form in a lot.
2. I give a vaccine prepared from lungs infected with CCPP by homogenising the pneumonic lung tissue (at about 2000 rpm in mixer/grinder), lightly centrifuging the suspension and then the supernatant mostly lipid and the bottom deposit, mostly fibrous tissue are discarded. The middle liquid portion is collected. It is diluted with some distilled water. The diluted fluid is filtered through fine steel filter and then through sterile muslin cloth. The filtrate is heated in hot water bath (not directly on flame). The temperature is watched over by immersed thermometer till it reaches 60°C. It is maintained at 60°C for about 15 minutes and then slowly raised up to 70–72°C for a short-time (5 to 7 minutes) and then gradually cooled. The homogenate is centrifuged to remove deposited particles by centrifugation at 2000–2500 rpm. Antibiotics like Dicrysticine and Ceftriaxone and Ketoheal (Ketoconazole) as antifungal are added. This homogenate is used as vaccine at dose rate of 0.5 ml subcut. A safety test is done in 2 animals which should show thermal response of 2–3°F above preinjection temperature. The dose may be repeated after 6 months.

The disease can be diagnosed best by postmortem. Pneumonic grayish red or red consolidated lung covered with fibrinous exudates is the main lesion. Fever, purulent nasal discharge and anorexia are seen.

In areas when the disease is endemic , as in Gujarat, Rajasthan and Maharastra, I repeat tiamutin again 1 month after arrival of new lot.

Treatment

1. Orally tiamutin (Vetmulin 80%) is given at the rate of 20 mg per kg BW. Double of preventive dose for 3 to 5 days. "Avitia" (of Brihans) can also be used. TROX

of Virbac also contains Tylosin tartrate soluble powder. It may be given orally at the rate of 10 mg/kg BW orally in water or with jaggery.

2. Tylan 200 injection can be given in sheep and goats at the rate of 17 mg/kg injection IM. Oxytetracyclin LA can also be given to supplement Tiamutin.

3. *Breathease:* A preparation of Neospark co. is good to reduce inflammation and to stimulate immunity. Available in 100 ml bottles. Give 1–2 ml per sheep and goat orally, in water.

4. Megludyne (of VIRBAC can also be injected. 1.1 to 2.2 mg/kg/BW by IM/IV route for 3 to 5 days or 1–2 ml Megludyne per 45 kg BW as slow injection. It can be used in dogs, horses, camel and pigs.

5. Tolfine 8% (Vetoquinol product) can be injected subcut at the rate of 1 ml for 40 kg BW in all respiratory diseases. It is a NSAID.

Homoeopathic

Belladonna 1000 as above till the animal recovers.—1/4 teaspoonful, evening/afternoon

Tylan 200 is imported and marketed in India by Eli lily Asia Inc., India branch office. Ravshan, 1st floor Brunton road, Banglore. 560025 INDIA. (Imported from Northern Ireland)

Azee 500: It is Azythromycin injection by Cipla. It is used within 24 hours after it is dissolved in 5 ml diluent supplied with injection. The dissolved drug contains 100 mg per ml. In adult goat or sheep (about 30–35 kg/BW) half of the fluid 2.5 ml is injected IV and the remaining subcut before 24 hours. This may be followed by 250 mg oral dose (tablet) per day for 3 to 5 days.

▓ MAEDI

Maedi is a chronic, progressive pneumonia mainly of sheep but also seen in less severe form in goats. It has been recorded from Uttaranchal, UP and northern states. (Chauhan, HVS and Singh CM, 1970, British Vet J, 126:364).

Etiology: Non-oncogenic ovine retrovirus of subfamily Lentivirinae. This virus also produces a brain disease called VISNA but I have never recorded Visna in the brain examined. Disease spreads by air, water, infected milk and *in utero*.

Symptoms: The disease progresses slowly for months and results in respiratory distress particularly on long movement. There is loss of condition, weakness and death, in sheep or goats above 1 year age.

Pathology: Grossly the affected lungs remain inflated large, "rubbery" in consistency and grayish pink in colour. I have developed a field test for field diagnosis. If the surface of the affected lung is swabbed with glacial acetic acid then white, raised, sago like nodules are seen under the pleura. These represent histological formation of lymphoid nodules along with interstitial pneumonia which is the cause of "Rubbery" rather than spongy lungs.

Serodiagnosis: Agar gel precipitation test (AGPT) and ELISA test are used. Eradication is possible by culling seropositive of animals for which annual or better six monthly tests are done. Eradication is expensive. Newly introduced animals have to be tested before accepting in the flock.

Treatment: Not possible. Slaughter is the only step left.

◼ JAAGSIEKTE (OVINE PULMONARY ADENOMA OR PULMONARY ADENOMATOSIS)

It was called 'driving sickness' because like maedi more pronounced respiratory distress is seen after long walk in sheep.

Etiology

Jaagsiekte betaretrovirus.

Epidemiology

It is a worldwide disease of sheep with occasional mild cases in goats.

Histopathology

Lungs show patches of nodules along with satellite nodules, which histologically look like alveolar adenoma.

Treatment

Not possible.

◼ NONSPECIFIC PNEUMONIA

Cattle

1. *Mannheimia haemolytica* and *P. multocida* with parainfluenza virus (p3)
2. Parainfluenza 3 adenovirus 1 and 2
3. Chlamydia species
4. *Mycoplasma bovis* and *Mycoplasma californicum*
5. *Mycoplasma mycoides* causes contagious bovine pleuropneumonia.
6. Infection bovine rhinotracheitis (IBR) virus
7. Fog fever or epidemic acute interstitial pneumonia
8. Verminous pneumonia
9. Dusty feed rhinotracheitis.

◼ INFECTIONS CAUSED BY MYCOPLASMA CAPRINE AND OVINE CONTAGIOUS OPHTHALMIA (KERATOCONJUNCTIVITIS)

Etiology

Mycoplasma Conjunctivae: Infection occurs more by contact particularly in summer due to dusty winds.

Symptoms

Inflammation, redness of conjunctiva and flow of tears from eyes. Simillar to conjunctivitis is also produced by *M. arginini, M. capricolum, Mycoplasma mycoides* species and Rickettsial organisms, *Rupricapra rupricapae.*

Hosts

Sheep, goats and less severe in lambs and goats affecting about 10–12% of a flock. Recovery in 3 to 4 days.

Treatment

Injection of long-acting oxytetracycline (Oxy LA) a single injection along with ointment of cloxacillin helps in recovery in a week or more. Other eardrops such as

Otocinpet, Pomisol, and Ciprofloxacin can also be used. Otocin pet is quite good being bactericidal, anti-inflammatory and antiallergic (Pet Mankind product).

■ MYCOPLASMA ARTHRITIS IN CATTLE

Mycoplasma alklescens and *M. bovis* may produce polyarthritis with swelling of large joints of legs, lameness and slight fever. This disease is not important for India hence only a passing information is given here.

Treatment can be done with Tylosin as described under CCPP and also Enrofloxacin, but Tylosin is the best.

■ CONTAGIOUS AGALACTIA IN GOATS AND SHEEP

Contagious agalactia should be called a triad of mastitis arthritis and conjunctivitis (MAC disease) caused by *Mycoplasma agalactiae*, *M. mycoides* and *M. capricolum*.

Epidemiology

The disese is endemic including, India, middle east Asia and Australia.

Symptoms

There is fever, septicaemia, mastitis, arthritis and conjunctivitis. There is complete agalactia with many abscesses forming in udder. Organisms are abundant in milk and persist for months and years.

Diagnosis

PCR, CFT or ELISA tests can be done.

Treatment

Enrofloxacin, tylosin and tetracycline are used. I use a autogenous vaccine in CCPP. The same method hopefully should work but I have not come across this disease so far.

■ CONTAGIOUS BOVINE PLEUROPNEUMONIA (CBPP)

This is not an important disease in most parts of India hence a summary about the disease is given.

Etiology

Mycoplasma mycoides subspecies mycoides. It is not a common and important disease. There is no vaccine and no reputed drug for treatment in allopathic.

Treat with Tiamutin preparations as mentioned under contagious caprine pleuropneumonia. Also, give homoeopathy: Silicia 200 (homoeopathic) 1/2 tea-spoonful every 4th day.

Symptoms

"Carriers" are the source of infection mainly by inhalation of infective droplets of expired air of carrier or diseased cattle.

In acute form: There is high fever of about 105°F respiratory distress, grunting sound, oedematous swelling of throat and dewlap.

Subacute and chronic form: Respiratory distress chronic cough and anorexia due to toxaemia.

Diagnosis

1. Presence of 'marbled' appearance of affected lung due to thickened septae of the lungs and presence of necrotic sequestra of 1 to several centimetre diameter. Fibrinous pleurisy is also seen.
2. *Laboratory tests:* PCR , histopathology and FAT are used.

Control

1. Slaughter of sick animals
2. Vaccination (not in India) with live attenuated strains.

Treatments

Mycoplasma do not have cell wall hence B-lactam is useless, other antibiotics useful are erythromycin, tylosin, oxytetracyclin (LA), and chloramphenicol.

Fluxivet (contains Flunixin 50 mg/ml a product of Carus Laboratories Pvt Ltd. It is to be used as stated below:

Species	Indications	Dose	Administration	Frequency
Cattle	Acute respiratory disease	2 ml/45 kg 1 ml/ 45 kg BW	IM or IV	One or two doses (divided) at 12 hours, packing 20. 50, and 100
Sheep	Acute coliform mastitis			
Goats	Fever			
Camel	Diarrhoea			
Dogs	Muscle diseases/infection			

▓ GOAT POX

Etiology

Capripox virus (Variola capra) and sheep pox virus affect goats and sheep respectively but recombination may occur.

Epidemiology

Recorded in India, very virulent strain was found by me in Bihar and eastern India, particularly in Black Bengal goats. It is highly contagious, viremic disease which spreads fast by air, contact and mosquitoes (which bite in hairless parts).

A soluble noninfectics antigen has been developed by Rao TVS and Bandhopadhyay SK (2000) Animal Health Rev, 1: 127). This can be obtained by post. AGPT test is easy to perform and confirms the diagnosis besides. ELISA test is also used.

Treatment

There is no specific treatment. Only preventive vaccination is possible. The vaccine is available in most of the biological products institutes.

Sheep Pox Vaccine

From Institute of Animal Health and Veterinary Biologicals, Hebbal, Bangalore 560024. Email: director_iahvb@dataone.in, Phone 08043411502.

Goat pox and sheep pox vaccine: from Indian Veterinary Research Institute, Izatnagar, Bareilley, UP.

Hester Biosciences Ltd produces live IP (Uttarakashi strain) against goat pox, it is derived from verocell culture. This vaccine is recommended for vaccination in 4 month and older goats. It is advised to vaccinate after kidding season and before breeding season. Freeze dried vials are available in dose of 25, 50, and 100. Like PPR. Chilled diluent (below 8°C) is mixed. Small quantity of diluent is added into the vial, powder is dissolved, vaccine is taken out by syringe and mixed with the remaining chilled diluent (25 ml or 50 ml or 100 ml) and mixed. One millilitre of dissolved vaccine is injected subcutaneously into neck with sterile syringe and needle.

Symptoms and Lesions

Pox lesions in the form of raised nodules are found mainly in the hairless parts of body (face, ears, thighs, tail, etc). The disease spreads fast to affect more than 75% animals with mortality going as high as 80–85%. Lungs show white raised solid nodules (sometimes also in kidney) surrounded by congestion. Nodules are about 5 mm to 1.5 cm in diameter. There is viremia and high fever.

Treatment

Vaccination is the most desirable step. Otherwise only symptomatic treatment without much results are the only alternatives.

Comparison of Nonspecific Pneumonia

Differential Diagnosis Chart of Nonspecific Pneumonia (calves and other ruminants).

Agents	Symptoms	History	Treatment
1. Mannheimia haemolytica + 2. *P. multocida* + PI 3 virus	Bronchopneumonia moderate dyspnoea fever, gargling sounds, cough, neutropenia with leukopenia	Transportation mixing of animals Epidemic form may or may not start soon on arrival but a week or 15 days later	1. As suggested for pasteurellosis 2. Best drug is 'Cobactan' of MSD containing Cefquinome sulphate (1 mg/kg) with Avil or Megludyne 3. Cur X (LA) 30 ml for 400 kg BW
3. Parainfluenza 3 (PI3) Virus	Acute pneumonia, as above but gargling sounds not heard, lymphopenia and leukopenia	Addition of new lot in a closed herd high morbidity and low mortality	1. Treatment to prevent secondary bacterial infections 2. Homoeopathic: Belladonna IM and Phosphorus 200
4. Chlamydial pneumonia: *Chlamydophila pneumoniae* affects cattle, sheep, goats and *Ch. psittaci* in pigs	As described for enzootic pneumonia, fever (39 to 42°C) respiratory distress. Occasionally diarrhoea, abortion in last trimester	Enters through latently infected new lot. Fever. Host usually 2-6 months old	1. Treatment to prevent secondary bacterial infections 2. homoeopathy as above

Contd...

Agents	Symptoms	History	Treatment
5. Infectious Bovine Rhinotracheitis virus (IBR). Cause is Bovine Herpes Virus-1 + PI3+ 6. Bovine coronavirus, etc.	Outbreak, dyspnoea, loud coughing, nasal discharge, nasal congestion ('pink nose'). Fever for 3 to 5 days, 1% mortality all age group affected Rectal temperature above 40 °C.	Infection enters through, grass, feed and water	1. No specific treatment 2. Homoeopathy as above 3. Symptomatic such as injections of 'Melonex', etc.
7. Dusty feed Rhinotracheitis dust inhaled through highly powdered, dusty feed	Severe coughing, serous nasal discharge, conjunctivitis with redness and watery discharge	Exposure to dusty feed	1. Recovery in 2 days after discontinuing dusty feed
8. Allergic summer or spring season rhinitis	Crop in flowering stage or wild grass in flowering stage. Seasonal autmn or summer occurance	Sneezing, mucous or mucopurulent discharge, rubs nose against wall or twigs, rubbing nose against solid objects; open mouth breathing	1. Antihistaminics like Avil or Cadistin (Zydus) IM injection 3–5 ml in large and 0.5 to 1 ml in small animals *Homoeopathic:* Apismel 200 ½ teaspoonful 3 times a day in water

PESTEDES PETITS RUMINANTS (PPR, GOAT PLAGUE)

It is the most important disease of goats and sheep mostly confined to Africa, Middle East, Asia and most parts of India.

Etiology

Morbillevirus (PPRV) belonging to lineage 1, 2, 3 and 4. Indian strain belongs to lineage 4. The virus is antigenically similar to rinderpest, distemper viruses and measles virus of humans.

Epidemiology

Infection occurs by inhalation or ingestion or water. Infection starts on mixing of healthy and diseased animals on farm or markets. Disease is more severe in goats than in sheep. Virus causes viremia.

Morbidity and Mortality

Mortality may be as high as 70 to 80% in goats and 10 to 30% in sheep, disease develops in all seasons but infection spreads fast on crowding or transportation in trucks. (through air and drinking water).

Symptoms

The disease is explosive as in case of rinderpest. Symptoms appear after 4 to 7 days after mixing with infected animal. High fever above 40 °C , dullness, loss of appetite, serous nasal discharge from nose and eyes, sneezing and coughing

After a few days diarrhoea as in rinderpest develops with watery or blood tinged faeces. Animals die within 5 to 6 days after onset of symptoms.

Important Lesions

Small necrotic spots and erosions develop on lateral surface and tips of tongue and lips but their absence does not rule out PPR. Most important lesions I have found are "Zebra" haemorrhagic lines in large intestine mainly near caeco colic junction and pneumonia (due to secondary bacterial or mycoplasmal infection), lymph nodes are enlarged.

Diagnosis

1. Sudden onset of fabrile disease, high mortality, history of mixing of animals
2. Agar gel precipitation test (AGPT)
3. *Virus neutralization test:* VNT is recognized for international sale and purchase
4. *ELISA:* Nasal secretions and buffy coat of blood of sick animals can be used as antigen for these tests.

Control

Good vaccines are available, such as Hesters PPR vaccine (96 strain): Live, freeze dried vaccine, supplied on purchase order under cold chain. Storage below 8°C but not in freezing chamber. For details contact www. Hester.in (Hester Bioscience Ltd, Pushpak, Level one, Panchvati circle, Motilal hirabhai road, Ahmedabad, Gujarat 380006, India: Doses 25, 50 and 100 dose vials with diluents). Vaccine is supplied at the farm/hospital.

Keep new stock in clean, quarantine. Vaccinate as early as possible in 4 months or older animals after 6 months (repeat)

PPR vaccine is also available from vaccine institute Hebbal Bangalore and from Indian Veterinary Research Institute, Izatnagar, Bareilly, UP, but these agencies do not supply vaccine at door step.

Precaution

1. If PPR is suspected, immediately remove clinically sick animals with higher body temperature away from the remaining flock.
2. Immediately vaccinate the healthy goats/sheep and wait for immunity to develop in about 14 days. Before this period remove the sick animals away to distant place away from healthy ones. Do not use a common drinking container because virus spreads fastest through water.

▓ BRUCELLOSIS (CATTLE)

Etiology

Brucella abortus

Hosts

Cattle of all ages, wild bisons, buffaloes, horses (localised), pigs and sheep (rarely with abortion) dogs (unsymtomatic), it causes "Undulating fever" in man with complication of chronic arthritis.

Mode of Action

Brucellosis is quite prevalent in some states of India (e.g. Gujarat). It is highly pathogenic and can produce infection orally, intact skin and conjunctiva. Source of organisms are pasture, aborted foetus, foetal membranes, infected calves (up to 4 to

6 months after calving by infected cow). Infected calves should not be used for breeding. Infection is a lesser threat for bulls, more if AI is used. Sexually immature cattle can also get infected.

Pathology

The bacteria localized in the lymph nodes all over the body and in the foetal mambranes of pregnant cows.

Diagnosis

1. Indirect ELISA (IELISA)
2. *Fluorescence Polarization Assay (FPA):* This is easy and portable method.
3. Rose Bengal Plate Test (RBPT): 1. Antigen for the test is available from Institute of Animal Health and Veterinary Biologicals, Hebbal, Bangalore 56002.
4. Brucella Abortus antigen for serum agglutination test is also available from Division of Biological Products, Indian Veterinary Research Institute, Izzatnagar, Bareilly. Method of test is given on the antigen bottle.
5. Card test
   Bovine Brucella Antibody Detection Kit (Scanvet) is a kit produced by Intas Pharmaceuticals Ltd, Ahmedabad, India. It is a lateral flow immunochromatographic method. The test plate has invisible test (T) and control (C) zones. For test serum or plasma of suspected animal (store 2 to 3°C) is used.

Method

1. Take out cassette and place it on a flat surface
2. Add by a dropper 1 drop of blood or 2 drops of serum or plasma to the empty vial. Shake the vial gently after adding 4 drops of assay diluents to the vial
3. Using a dropper add one drop of diluted mixture into the sample hole (S)
4. After the sample drop is completely absorbed, add 3 drops of assay diluents into the sample hole (S)
5. Wait for 10 to 20 minutes and take final results up to 20 minutes
6. Results
   a. It two lines are seen on the test plate then the sample is positive
   b. If only one red coloured line is seen on the test plate then the test is negative.

Assay Parameters:

Sensitivity	96.8 %	(Data based on comparison with Complement
Specificity	99.1%	Fixation Test (CFT) Terrestrial manual and
		Minimum Antibody Titre 120 IU/ml European
		commission directive 64/432/EEC, Annex C)

Prevention and Treatment: Brucella abortus cotton strain S 19 vaccine is used for control in infected herd. A vaccine is available from Hester Biosciences Ltd, Pushpak Level One, Panchvati Circle, Motilal Hirabhai Road, Ahmedabad, Gujarat 380006, www.hester.in, mail@hester.in, toll free number 18002332797. The vaccine is freeze-dried, to be diluted with diluent supplied with the vaccine and prepared as described for PPR vaccine. Store FD vaccine below 8°C.

Prophylactic vaccination is done in female calves between 3 and 6 months age as a single subcutaneous injection of 2 ml at middle of the neck.

■ BRUCELLA MELITENSIS INFECTION

Brucellosis caused by *Br. Melitensis* appears to be unrecorded in India. Goats and sheep suffer from the disease in countries of Asia hence caution to prevent entry of infection is necessary. Carrier animals (latent disease) may bring the disease into our country. Abortion generally occurs in the last two months of pregnancy. In humans, Br. Melitensis produces Malta fever or mediterranian fever. The organisms can also be used as an instrument of bioterrorism, by use of aerosol infection.

Treatment: May be attempted with tetracycline LA injections or Streptomycin injections.

Other causes of Infectious Abortions and their Differentiation

Disease	Observation	Treatment
Brucellosis	Abortions take place generally in last 3 months of pregnancy. After abortion, foul-smelling, slimy exulate comes out. Placenta looks leathery	(xxx) Not effective (see under Brucellos)
Trichomoniasis (Trichomonas protozoa)	Abortion occurs in first 2–4 months of pregnancy. The foetus abortion percentage is less (5–30%). Pyometra may develop. Exudates is clear and seromucous without smell. Flagellated protozoa are seen in hanging drop preparation	1. *Curacin-OZ (Vets Pharma):* 30–60 ml per horn daily for 3–5 days 2. *Griptol-N:* Oral liquid Levofloxacin + Ornidol; dose—10 ml per 40 kg BW for 3–4 days 3. Metacade injection (Realcade Life Co) IV/IV (5–25 mg/kg BW, 12 hourly
Leptospirosis (febrile disease)	Abortion occurs at around 6 months. Cotyledone becomes yellowish or brown. Dark ground examination will show motile snake-like leptospira	(xx) Dihydrostreptomycin injection (25 mg/kg BW IM is recommended). Inject dogs with Oxytetracyclin 20 mg/kg BW) for 5 days or Erythromycin (25 mg/kg BW IM daily for 5 days)
Vibriosis	Abortion at 5–6 months of pregnancy. Small red spots are seen on the placental surface with placental oedema	(o-x) No specific treatment but metronidazole may be tried or Curacin-OZ 30 ml in each horn may be tried, dimetritazole in bulls
Listeriosis	Abortion occurs mostly in the 7th month of pregnancy. Also, septicaemia may occur. Abortion rate is 100%	Injections of Chlortetracyclin 10 mg/kg IM for 5 days. Penicillin 44000 IU/kg BW, IM 7–14 days

■ SALMONELLOSIS (Paratyphoid Fever, Enteric Fever)

Salmonallosis affects all animal species, human beings and poultry. There are hundreds of species (more than 2000 serotypes) of Salmonella but only a few important ones are of practical, clinical importance.

S. typhimurium, S. duobulin in ruminants and horses; S. saintpaul, S. Enteritidis, Dublin, S. Newport and S. Cholerae suis in pigs.

Symptoms: Septicaemia with high fever in newborn ruminants, foals and pigs, generally below 4 months age; with enteritis and abortion in adults. Infection rate is around 10 to 15%. There is severe diarrhea and dehydration in young ones, with dry gangrene of tips, of ears or tail, etc. (occasional) and occasionally arthritis. 'Winter dysentery' in cattle.

Diagnosis: By culture and tests in laboratory.

Treatment: Furazolidone is still quite effective against most salmonella, e.g. Pesulin MFL bolus (Cadila).

Antimicrobials as Injections

Example: **Lykacetin (Alembic)** 2–4 mg/kg BW IV. or 20–30 mg/kg BW IM contents are chloramphenicol, 1, 2, and 3 g vials
Lykadin (Alembic) bolus: Contains Sulphadimidine
Dose: 1 to 2 bolus/50 kg BW.

Rocklow: Ofloxacin 1000 mg; ornidazole 1800 mg
It inhibits DNA gyrase hence bacterial death. Effective in diarrhoea and dysentery of unknown origin (Mfg by Kepler Vet. Mission Pvt Ltd, Ahemedabad)
Dose: 1 bolus/100 kg BW; 3–5 days

Oxy-LA (Zydus): Oxytetracyclin vial of 30 ml. Inject at the rate of 1 ml/10 kg BW as a single shot by IM route only; effective for 3–4 days.

Cflox-TZ (Intas): Ciprofloxacin (1.5 g) + Tinidazole (1 g), 1 bolus/300 kg BW for 3–5 days is extremely good.

For dehydration:
a. Dextrose saline injection to prevent dehydration and to provide energy. (Dextrose 25 % Claris Amanta, Nirlife or Realcade Cos)
b. ORS in water to prevent dehydration and electrolyte imbalance

For Fever:
Melonex (Intas) inj. or bolus (100 mg) is good
Melonex Plus: Meloxicam + paracetamol
Inflavet Plus (Virbac)—Meloxicam 100 mg + paracetamol (1.5 g) can be given 1 bolus/200 kg BW in case of Melonex plus.

▨ BACILLARY HAEMOGLOBINURIA

Cause: Bacteria *Clostridium haemolyticum* infection enters via contaminated food or water. The toxins produce haemolysis, haemoglobinuria (red water), acute anaemia and jaundice, arched back, initially high fever and grunting.

Treatment: Penicillin and tetracyclin in high doses. Iron, copper, cobalt containing mineral supplements before the animal dies in 1–2 days.

▨ FOOT ROT AND SOLE ULCERS

Infectious foot rot in sheep

Etiology: D. nodosus bacteria of variable virulence
Organism gets passed on from one infected sheep to another. It is commonly observed by me here in Surat, Gujarat. The main guideline is lameness, slow walking sheep at the tail end of the flock which show foot lesions.

Lesion: Inflammation at the margin of hoof and skin, which later spreads in interdigital area under the hoof into laminae. One and often all feet get infected particularly, in rainy season due to aggravation by mud, warm humid environment.

Age affected: Sheep of all ages are affected. Cattle also get affected with *D. nodosus*, with pitting, and separation at skin horn junction at the heel part.

Treatment: Dip the affected feet in any or more than one of the following dips:
1. 50% copper sulphate solution (easily available from any chemist shop, also known as "Neela thotha").
2. 5% formalin 5% means 5 parts of formalin to make to 100 parts (20 times water).
3. Zinc sulphate solution (10 to 20%).

Let the treated animal stand on dry floor for a few hours after treatment. The foot bath treatment may be repeated after a few days or a week till recovery.

ANTIBIOTICS

The organisms D nodosus are resistant to sulfa drugs but susceptible to penicillin, chloramphenicol erythromycin, tylosin tartrate, nitrofurazone.
1. Dicrysticines (Zydus) is one of the best medicine which is also cost effective. It contains penicillin and streptomycin. (contains Penicillin 650000 units of procaine and sod. Penicillin)
   Streptomycin 2.5 g/Dicrysticine DS contains double of these quantities. Dissolve in 15 ml water
   Inject: Large animals 2 ml/50 kg BW
         Small animals 1 ml/5 kg BW
   Paking: Box of 25 vials
2. Lixen (Virbac) contains Cephalexin—1 bolus per 150 kg BW
   Sheep—20 g powder sachet: in 100 ml water. Give orally in 8–10 sheep for 3–5 days
3. Oxytetracyclin injections
4. Apply ointments on foot: Lyramycin (Lyca) cream or Calendula (Homoeopathic cream) + Calendula 30 globules (8–10) 3 times a day for quick healing
5. Seftifur injection (Mankind) is also quite effective also Seftifur sodium (Merial)
   Does—1.1 to 2.2 mg/kg BW, IM or SC, for 3–5 days.

COCCIDIOSIS

Coccidia include many Eimeria and Isospora species. Important ones are:
- Cattle (calves) —*E. zuernii, E. bovis*
- Goats—*E. arloingi* and 12 other species
- Sheep: *E. arloingi* and 5 other
- Pigs: Eisospora sp.

Coccidia and Cryptosporidia: Goats are very commonly affected, overcrowding, poor hygiene, young age, moisture in shed, cold season help in outbreak. I recorded this in Hissar in goats of Animal Science College of Agricultural University without much symptoms but mortality in anaemic kids. Almost 100% kids may get infected mortality may range between 20 and 40%.

In calves coccidiosis is the third most important health problem in newborn calves.
Coccidiosis causes diarrhoea in 5 to 15 days old piglets, resulting in low weight gain

Life Cycle: The life cycle is direct. After schizonts forming in intestinal epithelium, large gametes form which destroy the host epithelium causing bleeding from caecum and colon.

Symptoms: Foul-smelling diarrhoea, sudden onset and presence or absence of blood. Severe straining with dysentery is quite characteristic. In long run, anaemia with pale mucosae may be seen.

In calves, "nervous form" may occur in about 40% calves in winter. In such cases, there is lateral recumbancy, convulsions and opisthotonos.

Diagnosis: A count of 5000 or more oocysts per gram of faeces is considered clinically significant (Fig. 3.2).

Treatment:
1. Sulphadimidine (Sulphamezathine) a) 140 mg/kg BW, orally for 3 days in calves and lambs. Zydus Sulphabolus 5 g and Entradin bolus (Sulphadimidine) 5 g bolus dose: 2 bolus per 50 kg BW.
2. Amprolium: 10 mg/kg BW orally for 5 days (Wockhardt + Merind, Zydus, Piya Pharma Cos)
3. Monensin: 2 mg/kg BW for 20 days in sheep and goat
   For prevention about 25% of the doses may be given in feed for 2 to 3 weeks after about 4 to 5 week age.

■ CRYPTOSPORIDIOSIS

Etiology: Protozoan parasites *Cryptosporidium parvum* and *C. andersoni*

Host: Newborn calves, goats, kids, lambs and piglets all over the world are affected. Mainly 1 to 4 weeks old calves are susceptible. In kids and lambs, mixed infection is usually seen. In pigs the infection is mostly asymptomatic.

Symptoms: Mild diarrhoea looking like malabsorption type. Adult mother is the source of infection or it can also spread from calf to calf. (Feed water, through rodents and cats).

Life cycle: Parasites are in the intestinal epithelium which damages the cell. The cause of diarrhoea probably is atrophy of villi in small intestine. Combined infection with rotavirus is common.

Diagnosis: For clinical diagnosis presence of 10 to the power 5 or 10 to the power 7 oocysts per ml of faeces are important. Oocysts are small—5 to 6 nm in diameter and are difficult to detect by ordinary light microscope. Detection is easy, by floatation (sugar or salt) method. Staining can be done by modified Ziehl-Neelson stain.

Treatment:
1. Hyperimmune bovine colostrums or our injections of bovine immunoglobulins plus colostrums feeding can reduce the severity of diarrhoea.
2. Homoeopathic medication with a mixture of 9 types of biochemical medicines given under the chapter of diarrhoea (Cholera mixture) can be very effective.
3. Helofuginon: Stenerol (Intervet product) will act against coccidian as well as cryptosporidia. It is fed at the rate of 3 ppm (500 g/tonne feed) or 5 g per day from 1 to 4 weeks.
4. Vetrfur—TL (Merial) Metronidazole 1000 mg. Furazolidone 500 mg for diarrhoea, dysentery and mixed bacterial or protozoal infections and calf scours. *Dose:* Large animals 4–6 bolus per day for 3–5 days; small animals 1–2 bolus/day for 3 to 5 days. (15–25 mg/kg/day, orally).

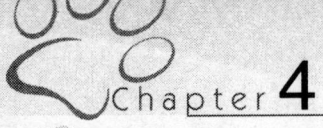

Chapter 4

Chronic Bacterial Diseases of Cattle, Sheep and Goat

The important chronic bacterial diseases of cattle, sheep, and goat are:
1. Tuberculosis: Not common and generally not treated
2. Johne's Disease of Paratuberculosis: Common in some areas
3. Actinomycosis
4. Actinobacillosis

■ BOVINE TUBERCULOSIS

Bovine tuberculosis even if detected, is not treated hence I am not dealing the details of this topic. One should know that tuberculin test can be done if suspected. Besides, lungs, respiratory tuberculous mastitis can also occur.

For tuberculin test a patch of skin of neck is shaved and 1 to 2 drops of 0.1 to 0.2 purified protein derivative (PPD) of *Mycobacterium bovis* is injected intradermally and the site of injection is marked with indelible marker pen. The thickness of skin at the site of injection is measured with a Vernier caliper on 0 day and also at 24–48 and 72 hours if the swelling becomes several times than on 0 day, the test is positive. False positive tests are seen in cases of avian tuberculosis, nocardia infection, etc. Tuberculin for this test is available from Indian Veterinary Research Institute, Izzatnagar, Bareilly.

■ JOHNE'S DISEASE—PARATUBERCULOSIS

This disease is caused by *Mycobacterium avium*, subspecies paratuberculosis ("MAP").

Symptoms

Chronic progressive diarrhoea which does not respond to treatment of any kind. There is emaciation and lastly, hide-bound condition. In sheep and goats also similar symptoms are seen. On postmortem, large and terminal part of small intestine shows thickening, corrugated appearance and presence of acid fast bacilli in the smears prepared from pinch of the thickend intestinal mucosa. Goats in Ranchi (Jharkhand) were affected more than sheep. The diseased animal has long incubation period and may excrete bacteria for 15–18 months. Clinical disease is precipitated by stress of malnutrition, pregnancy, etc. starting with loss of weight.

Generally, less than 5% of animals in a herd show symptoms. I detected infection in a goat flock of Ranchi Veterinary College in 1979–1980. The disease was eradicated by repeated Johnin test and segregation. Milk of the diseased cow is also a source of periodic excretion of the organisms. The bacteria survive for several months in soil. "Map" is also suspected to be associated with chronic enteritis called "Crohn's

Disease" in man and also detected in breast milk of some women. Only DNA of MAP is found in Crohn's disease affected intestine and not the a bacteria. (colitis). (Radostits et al. 2009, Vety Med, 9th Edn, p: 1021).

Diagnosis (Field) of Johne's Disease

1. Laboratory diagnosis by ELISA test is 85% sensitive.
2. All animals may be tested by Intradermal injection of 'Johnin', a ppd-like tuberculin. It is possibly available from Indian Veterinary Research Institute, Izzatnagar, Bareilly.

   Johnin antigen is injected intradermally in recommended dose and the skin thickness at the site of injection is measured before and after 24 hours or 36 hours. The thickness of skin should increase by 4 mm or more than the pre-test thickness.
3. *Fecal culture:* Fecal culture of *M. avium* paratuberculosis is considered as 100% reliable.

Treatment

Currently no line of treatment of JD is approved or reliable. MAP are more resistant to drugs than to *M. tuberculosis*. It is also expensive to try treatment.

Streptomycin can be injected at the dose rate of 50 mg/kg BW, IM, daily for several weeks and the animal may show slight recovery but may not be totally cured.

Minimise contact between young and old animals. Repeatedly test and eliminate the positive reactors at a few months intervals to keep the disease under control or for eradication.

ACTINOMYCOSIS (LUMPY JAW)

The veterinarians know about the cause and symptoms of actinomycosis hence details about the disease are skipped.

Cause

Actinomyces bovis.

Symptoms

A hard, immovable, tumorlike swelling on mandible (jawbone) or maxilla (facial bone). Later, small amount of pus is discharged from one or several openings. Growth takes 6–18 months to develop. Udder may also get affected by tumorlike nodular growths.

Treatment

Early treatment is more successful

Streptomycin 5 g/day/IM, 30 days.

Potassium or sodium iodate: 15–30 g dissolved in 250 to 300 ml distilled water; inject IV

Isoniazide 20 mg/kg BW for 100 days

Surgical débridement after exposure to liquid nitrogen

Homoeopathic: Silicia 200 1 teaspoonful and Hepar Sulph 200 one teaspoonful 3 times a day.

◼ ACTINOBACILLOSIS (WOODEN TONGUE)

Cause

Actinobacillus species (22 species)

But important in bovines is *A. lignieresii*. There is a granuloma formation in soft tissue such as tongue or subcutaneous tissue, causing hard, enlarged tongue protruding out of mouth.

Treatment

1. Give potassium iodide 10 g in jaggary for 10 days
2. Sod. Iodide: Dissolve 10 g to make 10% or 20% solution. Inject IV very slowly at the rate of 10 mg/120 kg BW; 1–2 days
3. Streptomycin 5 g/day/IM for 3–4 days
4. Mega Dox-N (Neospark): Doxycyclin + Neomycin; dose 10–20 mg/kg BW orally, 3–5 days.
5. *Homoeopathy:* For both Actinomycosis and Actinobacillosis, give Hepar Sulph 200 1 teaspoonful TDS and Silicia 200 1 teaspoonful TDS orally.

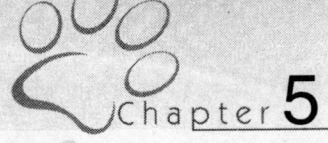

Chapter 5

Important Viral Diseases

■ FOOT AND MOUTH DISEASE (FMD, APHTHOUS FEVER)

Etiology

The disease is caused by Picorna virus. There are several strains, A, O, C, found in all countries.

Asia 1 and SAT 1 are found in Asia, including India.

Hosts: All cloven footed animals including pigs but cattle are the most important hosts.

Pathogenesis

Virus can enter by mouth or by air. First there is viraemia, then localisation in skin and tongue epithelium.

Symptoms

Fever, profuse salivation, later, vesicles form in the mouth and in the skin between and around hooves. Low mortality below 2% but high in calves and exotic animals (up to 20%).

Treatment

Only symptomatic for fever and antiseptic dressings. Disinfection of premises is done with any of the disinfectants dealt within a separate chapter.

Prevention

I have not seen any outbreak of FMD in 10 to 13 thousand cattle, sheep, and goats during 12 years of my service at Shri Surat Panjrapole, Surat, Gujarat.

First FMD Vaccine (Raksha FMD Vaccine) is prepared by Indian Immunologicals Hyderabad. Dose is 3 ml by subcutaneous root at the age of 3 weeks, booster injection at 4 months. The vaccine in endemic areas is repeated after 2 to 4 months. Later, vaccination may be done after every 6 months. It contains O, C, Asia 1 and A-22 types of virus. Subcut injection is given.

Second FMD vaccine is Baif Institute of Animal Health Vaccine. It is used in cattle, buffaloes, sheep and goats. Dose in calf is 10 ml and is 5 ml in sheep and goats.

Primary vaccination	Booster	Annual
Calves 6–8 week old 4–6 month old adult	4 month then 6 months	Every 6 months

Third FMD vaccine (Hoechst India Ltd). Dose: 10 ml in cattle and 5 ml in sheep and goats by subcut route.

Homoeopathic Treatment

1. Calendula spray "Woundwell" of SBL Pvt Ltd, e-mail: care@sblglobal.in; website: www.sbl.sblglobal.in
2. Calendula ointment of any company to be applied on the wound and ulcers (very important). This homoeopathic drug not only promotes healing but also prevents infection.
3. *Calendula 30 liquid:* Give 1/2 teaspoonful per animal twice daily (very important).
4. If large number of cattle are affected, then Calendula 30 liquid may be added in drinking water at the rate of 1 teaspoonful per 25 animals, morning and evening.
5. Liquid feed supplement such as 'Protin C' of Hester Co—the liquid is available in container of 170 ml, 1*l*, 2*l*, and 5*l*. Dose is 100 ml daily/animal for 10 days besides other soft food like gruel in milk, soya bean chunks soaked in water, etc.
6. 'Unixin' by IV or IM injection (20 ml package) at the rate of 1 ml (2 mg) per 50 kg BW for analgesic and antipyretic effect. Dose is 1.1 mg/kg BW by IV/IM route.
7. *Topicure SG:* (Natural Remedies): It is a herbal spray for ulcers in mouth, including FMD. It is available as a can of 100 ml. This may be used along with Calendula 30 (homoeopathic), 1/2 teaspoonful in water for fast healing.

■ RINDERPEST (CATTLE PLAGUE)

This disease was the biggest cause of losses of cattle which was one of the foremost cause to establish Imperial Veterinary Research Institute, now Indian Veterinary Research Institute of Bareilly, UP and the first veterinary school (1762) in Lyon, France. In india, the disease appears to be eradicated under Global Rinderpest Eradication Programme (GREP). I worked in GREP as a veterinary surgeon in the year 1959 to 1962.

Etiology

Cause of Rinderpest is *Morbilli* virus called rinderpest virus, antigenically similar to PPR virus, distemper viruses.

Mode of Infection

Orally or by inhalation, biting flies and ticks.

Symptoms

Similar to those described for PPR. India has been free from Rinderpest since 1990, but the disease was recorded in Pakistan in 2000–2002, hence need to be careful. Morbidity is 100% and mortality is around 50%.

Hosts: Cattle, buffaloes (less severe) rarely in pigs, sheep and goats.

Diagnostic Tests

Similar to those described for PPR histologically formation of syncytial giant cells in the epithelial cells of erosions of tongue. Basophilic intranuclear inclusion bodies are seen in smears of erosions.

Treatment

Rabbit adopted vaccine is safe for cattle including exotic breeds. Rinderpest appears to have been recorded in India up to 1991. (Datta, J. et al. 1991, Indian Vet J, 105: 20). Chicken embryo adopted vaccine is also used in some countries. Tissue culture vaccine is available in India. Dose is 1 ml SC injection. Verocell adopted vaccine is best for India (Chatterjee et al. IVJ 70.695). The measles vaccine protects calves against rinderpest when ordinary rinderpest vaccines are ineffective (Provost, A, et al. Rev Elev Med Vet. Pays. Trop, 1986, 21: 14 S)

▩ BLUE TONGUE (BTV) (SORE MUZZLE)

Host: Sheep

Etiology

Orbi virus of Reoviridae family. There ar 24 antigenic types. This virus is resistant to heat drying and even disinfection hence post outbreak care is to be taken. This virus may survive for 7 years.

Epidemiology

All tropical and subtropical countries including India are affected (almost all states from J and K to Tamilnadu and Haryana, MP to West Bengal).

Mode of Infection

Most common mode of BTV spread is through bites of 1400 species of culicoides species of mosquitoes which mostly bite at night, specially in wet, irrigated or canal areas. Sheep ticks can also transfer the infection mechanically or by blood. Cattle act as reservoir of virus. Five serotypes cause the disease commonly although a dozen or more serotypes exist (1 to 24).

Host: Clinical disease only in sheep. Cattle and goats are carriers.

Pathogenesis and Symptoms

The virus attached to RBCs produces viremia. They damage the endothelium of blood vessels, resulting in bleeding in tongue, uterus, causing abortion. Mortality varies from strain to strain and may be 2 to 3% or 50 to 75%. Infection does not protect from other strains (is strain specific). Symptoms are seen in more than one year old sheep these symptoms are:
1. High fever and loss of appetite.
2. Serous nasal discharge which later becomes blood tinged. Breathing difficulty and snoring.
3. Swelling and congestion of lips, tongue, mucosa of mouth, nose, muzzles and foul smell from mouth.
4. Hoof and skin junctions (corona) are congested and swollen.
5. Muscular damage results in stiff gait, weakness, and arching of back (opisthotonos).
6. Death occurs due to failure of respiration (lungs fail due to haemorrhages and pneumonia).

Diagnosis

Easiest is AGPT test. The provided antigen is available. Fluorescent antibody test (FAT)—this is better done after passage into chick embryos using infected RBCs.

Treatment

No treatment except symptomatic.

Control:
1. Control of mosquitoes, particularly at night.

2. *Vaccination:* In India, 18 serotypes exist, hence polyvalent vaccine is needed. Institute of Animal Health and Veterinary Biological, Hebbel, Bangalore have started commercial production of inactivated BTV vaccine but on trial basis. Website: www.iahvb.com, e-mail: director_iahvb@dataone.in, Phone 23411502, 23411661

VIRAL DISEASES OF PETS

RABIES

Signs

Disease or symptoms may develop after 2 weeks to several months post bite. Nearer the place of bite to brain, shorter will be the incubation time and vice versa.

Cattle may show strange behaviour such as bellowing, uncoordinated movement, frothing in mouth, drooling of saliva, recumbancy and death in less than a week. Somewhat similar signs are seen in sheep and goats.

Infection

Rabid dogs, rabid mongoose, jackals, etc. introduce infection in dogs and ruminants.

Etiology

The virus belongs to Lyssavirus genus and Rhabdoviridae family. It is a segmented RNA virus. Classical Rabies virus (RABV) occurs worldwide.

Mode of Infection

Infection is almost always by bite of an infected animal although inhalation may produce infection (not proven but suspected).

Symptoms

Post bite (average) incubation period in calves: 15 days. Duration of disease is less than 4 days.

Post bite incubation period in sheep: 10 days. Duration of the disease is less than 3.5 days.

Post bite incubation period in dogs: up to 2 weeks. Death after 1onset of symptoms: 4 to 7 days

Virus is richest in saliva, milk and foetus but not in blood.

The disease is always fatal.

Initially, there is melancholic behaviour like attempt to bite flies, yawning, bellowing in cattle, incoordination, drooling of saliva, recumbancy and death.

In furious form, there is hypersensitivity and irritability with tendency to bite without provocation. In sheep, there may be wool pulling. The terminal form is paralytic with paralysis and death. After paralysis of hind quarters, paralysis of anus and most constant is drooling of saliva.

Control and treatment

Prevention of rabies is the most important part of pet management and also of rearing cattle and horses. Vaccines are listed below:

1. *Rabigen:* Manufactured by Virbac which achieves high VNA titer which contains VP12 strain of rabies virus in aluminium hydroxide gel. (single dose 1 ml vial and 10 ml vial).

Use: For active immunization of dogs, cats, cattle, horses, and other mammals, also for post bite prophylaxis

Dosage: 1 ml dose whatever the species, age breed, sex and weight (SC).

2. Raksharab Rabies vaccine: Produced by Indian Immunologicals. Contains CVS strain.
   Use: For immunization and post bite prophylasis in dogs and cats.
   Dose: 1 ml by SC or IM route.
   Available as 1, 5 and 10 ml vials
   Time: Prophylactic injection is given at 3 months age. Primary vaccination may be given (optional) below 3 months age. Immunity lasts for 3 years. Annual vaccination may be done in endemic areas.
   Post bite vaccination: 0 day (as soon as possible) after bite, 3rd, 7th, 14th and 28th days.

3. Rabvac 3: Manufactured by Pfizer. It contains killed rabies virus (Street Alabama Dufferin strain).
   Use: Dogs, cats, and horses. Immunity duration is 3 years in dogs and cats and 1 year in horses.
   Dose: 1 ml SC or IM at 3 month or later age.

4. Canishot RV-F: Intas product. Killed (KC) rabies vaccine. Single does vial of 1 ml.
   Dose: Initial vaccination at 3–4 months age booster vaccination, yearly. SC or IM injection of single dose with diluents.

5. Rabivac-DHPPL: Product of MSD. It contains attenuated Pasteur RIV strain absorbed on aluminium phosphate
   Use: In dogs, cats, cattle, sheep, goats and horses.
   Dose: 1 ml as SC or IM injection.
   One box contains 1 ml × 10 vials or 10 ml × 10 vials.

6. Nobivac (puppy)—1 ml (MSD) single dose.

7. Nobivac RL (MSD): Contains Rabies strain mentioned above with *Leptospira icterohaemorrhagiae*; Lepto. Canicola inactivated.
   Use: 1 ml SC injection in dogs from 8 weeks onward. Packing of 1 ml × 10 vials
   To reduce pain and fever after injection injection of 'Fevnil', a combination of Nimesulide 100 mg and paracetamol 150 mg. Homoeopathic medicine Aconite 30 (5–6 globules orally or 1 drop in water) may be given.

8. Biocan R is a vaccine against rabies, target animals are dogs and cats. The animals are vaccinated from three months of age. The protective immunity starts 14 days after immunization. The animals first vaccinated at the age of 3 to 12 months must be re-vaccinated one year after the first application of the vaccine. The re-vaccination performed one year after the first vaccination shall protect the animals from rabies for a minimum period of 2 years.
   Post bite schedule: for the attacked animals, vaccinations of 1 ml should be applied on the 1st, 3rd, and 7th day after bite.

9. Defensor (injection 10 ml): A vaccine for dogs and cats 3 months of age or older. It is composed of killed rabies virus.
   Dosage: Aseptically administer 1 ml SC or IM at 3 month or age or older. Annual revaccination with a single dose is recommended.

10. *Rabvac 3:* Composed of killed rabies virus (Street Alabama Dufferin (SAD) strain).
    Indications: For dogs, cats, and horses. The vaccine provides 3 years of immunity for dogs and cats and a one year duration of immunity for horses. Dosage: Inject 1 ml SC or IM at 3 months or older in dogs and cats. Revaccinate one year later

and every 3 years thereafter. 2 ml dose SC or IM is to be given to horses 3 months or age or older. Revaccinate annually thereafter.
11. Rabivac Vet (10 ml vial of Brilliant Co).

Wound Toileting – Post Bite Management

Action
Wash the wound caused due to bite with running tap water
Gentle washing with soap or detergent and flushing the wound with running water for 10 minutes
After thorough washing and drying the wound, apply antiseptics (povidone iodine/ chlorhexidine gluconate/ cetrimide solution)

Points to be remembered

Don'ts	Reason/purpose
Touching the bite wound with bare hand	Increase in risk of exposure
Cauterization of the bite wound	Can leave a very bad scar and does not help in providing any additional advantage over the wound dressing
Application of irritants (chillies, oil, turmeric, lime, salt, etc.)	Can cause additional damage, delay the healing process. Stick to medical advise only.
Suturing of the wound	Makes the wound more susceptible to the entry of the virus.
Injection of tetanus toxoid	If unavoidable, apply minimum loose sutures after wound toileting and infiltration of rabies immunoglobulins
Injection of antibiotics	To prevent tetanus due to contamination of the bite wound with *Cl. Tetani* spores
	To prevent sepsis of the wound due to secondary bacterial infection

Special Circumstances

Circumstances	Do's/Don'ts
Pregnancy, lactation, infancy, old age, and concurrent illness	No contraindications for rabies postexposure prophylaxis in the event of an exposure
Immunocompromised state (HIV/ AIDS -CD4: less than 200 counts)	*Category II Bite:* Administer rabies immunoglobulin in addition to postexposure vaccination
	Estimation of antibody titre: If the facilities are available, estimation should be done 10 days after the completion of the course of vaccination
Human-to-human transmission	No risk (documented few cases resulting from organ transplant)
	People who have been exposed closely to the secretions of a patient with rabies may be offered PEP as a precautionary measure

Exposure to Rabies Infection

There is no need for human or doctor's vaccination if:
1. Only clothes have been torn without injury to skin
2. If the dog is normal, healthy and shows no sign of disease up to 10 days post bite.
   Class III or severe exposure: This is quite risky and includes all bites on neck and above.

According to WHO recommendations, antirabic sera and its globulin fraction should be injected in all cases of Class III exposure.

For prevention and treatment of rabies, a new Merinex inactivated rabies virus vaccine has been developed in France. It is a betapropiolectone inactivated rabies virus vaccine made from virus grown in beta/human diploid cell culture.

Take care before using antirabic vaccine:
1. The vaccine should be stored at 2–5°C temperature for less than 6 months in refrigerator and not at room temperature even if the expiry date is not over
2. Do not use the vaccine beyond expiry date.
3. Vaccine should never be exposed to sunlight.
4. Less fatty area should be selected for vaccination.

OTHER VIRUS DISEASES OF DOGS AND CATS

CANINE DISTEMPER

Distemper is acute, febrile disease of dogs. Often it is fatal. It affects young dogs, mainly 2 months to 1 year old, and mature dogs occasionally.

Cause

Morbillivirus

Mode of infection

By direct or indirect contact.

Symptoms

Fever for 3 to 4 days. Second febril response occurs after 8 to 12 days due to secondary bacterial infection, usually due to bacterial bronchopneumonia (Biphasic fever). Newborn pups may die due to myocarditis.

"Old dog encephalitis" is a chronic form of distemper. This is characterised by convulsions and incoordinated movement.

Summary of symptoms are biphasic fever; dentition age is more likely to be affected. There is watery discharge from eyes, sluggishness, later mucous and pus may be discharged from eyes and nose; bronchopneumonia; haemorrhagic gastroenteritis and diarrhoea; great loss of body weight, opacity of cornea; recovery or death in 29 days. Chronic cases may continue up to 12 weeks.

Diagnosis

Scanvet: Canine distempter antigen detection kit for diagnosis in suspected cases—contains antigen detection test cassette along with diluents, dropper, and sterile swab.

Scanvet: Canine Parvovirus Test Kit: Each kit contains detection test cassette with assey diluents, dropper, and sterile swab.

Vaccines

1. Venguard Plus 5 L4 Vaccine (Pfizer product): This is a vaccine to protect against distemper (CDV) canine adeno (CAV1 AND CAV2), canine Parvo (PiV), CPV and CPV2C and Leptospirosis (9 in 1 by Zoetis, USA: for 6 weeks or older dogs
   Dose: 1 ml SC by dissolving in diluents. *Leptospira grippotyphosa, L. icterohaemorrhagiae,* and *L. pomona* infections are also prevented. Apploximate cost is ₹ 800. Storage

at 2 to 7°C but never freeze. Burn all containers. If anaphylactic reaction takes place, inject epinephrine or similar antiallergens. Contact Zoetis (855) 424-7349 (USA). www.zoetisus.com or say hellow to 24/7 online shopping from Zoetis.

2. *Canishot K 3 (Intas):* Canine distemper, canine adenovirus-2, canine parvovirus, canine parainfluenza virus vaccine.
   Adenovirus include: Canine hepatitis, respiratory diseases.
   Dose: 1st: 6–7 weeks old. Sigle dose vial + diluent
   2nd: at 8–9 weeks
   3rd: 11–14 weeks
   Booster: Once annually SC

3. *Canigen DHP Vaccine (Virbac):* The vaccine contains live freeze dried fraction (one dose) canine distemper virus. Dissolve vaccine in diluent and inject by SC or IM route in puppies at 6 weeks age, followed by two injections of DHPP/L, one at 8 weeks and second at 12 weeks age. (see DHPPL under Leptospirosis).
   Protects against: Canine distemper virus (CPV)
   Canine adenovirus type 2 (CAV2), hepatitis virus

■ CANINE PARVOVIRUS

Packing: 1 ml × 10 vials with 10 vials diluents

1. *Canigen DHPPiL vaccine (Virbac):* Freeze–dried single dose. contains CDV, adenovirus (hepatitis), parvovirus, canine parainfluenza virus, canadenovirus, Leptospira, *L. icterohaemorrhagiae:* Age of immunisation is 8 weeks.

2. *Dosage:* Dissolve freeze-dried powder with liquid fraction. Inject one dose DHPPi/L by SC or IM route. Each box contains 25 single doses of DHPPi/L 25 vials of Canigen-L (Leptospira).
   Biocan DHPPI injection: BIOVETA (Netherlands) is a live vaccine against:
   a. Canine distemper (CDV)
   b. Inectious canine hepatitis (CAV1)
   c. Laryngotracheitis (CAV-2)
   d. Parvovirus (CPV-2; canine parvovirus enteritis)
   e. Parainfluenza (CPIV-2) in dogs.
   Dose: Dose is 1 ml regardless of age or weight or breed 1st injection in 6th week of age.
   Route: SC, preferably behind the shoulders.
   Storage: 2 to 8°C. When diluted, the vaccine should be injected immediately. See expiry date.
   No adverse reaction. Do not inject in dogs having fever.
   Puppy age:
   • 5–6 weeks
   • 7–8 weeks
   • 8–10 weeks—DHPPI + Leptospira
   • 12–16 weeks—DHPPI-LR
   Annual revaccination: DHPPI + LR
   Imported and marketed by Intervet India Pvt Ltd S no 136, Build-3, 3A +4 C, Warehouse Briahnagar, Office Pune Nagar Road
   Wagholi 412207 Dist, Pune

Pfizer Vaccines (Combined)
a. Vanguard 5 L (conventional polyvalent vaccine)

Indications: Provides protection against following viral diseases of dogs: 1. Canine distemper virus, 2. Canine parvovirus virus, 3. Canine parinfluenza virus, 4. Canine adenovirus type II, 5. *L canicola*, 6. *L. icterohaemorhaerrhagiae*.

Dosage: General direction: Vaccination of healthy dogs is recommended. Aseptically rehydrate the freeze dried vaccine with the liquid bacterin provided. Shake well and administer 1 ml SC or IV. Primary vaccination at 6 weeks age for healthy dogs followed by 2 booster doses administered 3–4 weeks apart. If vaccinated before the age of 4 months, they should be revaccinated with a single dose upon reaching 4 months of age.

Revaccination: Annual revaccination with single dose is recommended.
b. Vanguard Plus 5CVL (High titer low passage polyvalent vaccine).

Indications: Provides protection against the following diseases of dogs. 1. Canine distemper virus, 2. Canine parvovirus virus, 3. Canine parinfluenza virus, 4. Canine adenovirus type II, 5. Canine corona virus, 6. *L. canicola*, 7. *L. icterohaemohaerrhagia*.

Dosage: General direction: Vaccination of healthy dogs is recommended. Aseptically rehydrate the freeze dried vaccine with the liquid corona virus diluents. Shake well and administer 1 ml SC or IV. Healthy dogs at 6 weeks age or older should receive 3 doses, each administered 3 weeks apart. If vaccinated for the first time at 10–12 weeks of age, later only 2 vaccinations 3–4 weeks apart need be given.

Revaccination: Annual revaccination with single dose is recommended.
c. Vanguard CV (killed corona virus vaccine), zoetis product.

Indications provides protection against corona virus infection in dogs, which is the second most common cause of viral gastroenteritis in dogs.
Dosage: Healthy dogs 6 weeks of age or older should receive 3 doses, each administered 3 weeks apart.

Revaccination: Annual revaccination with single dose is recommended.
d. Durammune Max 5/4L (Polyvalent vaccine), Boehringer Ingelheim product, Canada.

Indications: Provides protection against: 1. Canine distemper virus, 2. Canine parvovirus, 3. Canine influenza virus, 4. Canine adenovirus type II, 5. *Leptospira canicola*, 6. *L. icterohaemohaerrhagiae*, 7. *Leptospira pomona* (seven in one)

Dosage: Aseptically rehydrate Duramune max 5 with Leptospira bacterial extract. Administer 1 ml dose SC. Primary vaccination should start at or about 6 weeks of age. Puppies should be revaccinated every 2 to 3 weeks until 12 weeks of age. All pups over 12 weeks of age should initially receive one dose of Duramune Max 5/4L and a second dose 2 to 3 weeks later. Annual revaccination with one dose is recommended.
e. Duramune Max 5 CVK/4L (polyvalent vaccine)

Indications: Provides protection against: 1. Canine distemper virus, 2. Canine parvovirus, 3. Canine parinfluenza virus, 4. Canine adenovirus type II, 5. *Leptospira canicola*, 6. *L. icterohaemohaerrhagiae*, 7. *Leptospira pomona*, 8. *Leptospira grippotyphosa* 9. Canine corona virus (9-in-one).

Dosage: Aseptically rehydrate duramune Max 5 CVK/4L with corona virus diluent. Administer 1 ml dose SC. Primary vaccination should start at or about

6 weeks of age. Puppies should be revaccinated every 2 to 3 weeks until 12 weeks of age. All pups over 12 weeks of age should initially receive one dose of Duramune Max 5 CVK/4L and a second dose 2 to 3 weeks later. Annual revaccination with one dose is recommended.

DISEASES CAUSED BY ADENOVIRUS

Two canine diseases caused by adenovirus (only of clinical value) are mentioned below:

Genus: Mastadenovirus:

Virus	*Disease*
i. Canine adenovirus 1	Infectious canine hepatitis
ii. Canine adenovirus 2	Upper respiratory tract infection in dogs

CANINE VIRAL HEPATITIS (RUBARTH DISEASE)

Both the above viruses are antigenically related

Infection: Contamination of food, water or air by urine, faeces or saliva of the diseased dog. Urine contains virus for about 4 weeks postinfection.

Symptoms: The disease begins with dullness, loss of interest, loss of appetite, vomiting, diarrhoea, fever (around 104°F), abdominal pain and occasionally oedema of ventral parts of the body (head, neck and abdomen). Urine may show albumin. Eyes may develop severe conjunctivitis, opacity of cornea, and high SGOT, SGPT in blood.

Prolonged bleeding time (BT) and clotting time (CT) are seen along with lymphocytosis.

CANINE LARYNGOTRACHEITIS

In canine adenovirus type 2 infection laryngotracheitis and sometimes pneumonia is seen. In liver cells presence of intranuclear inclusion bodies is typical and diagnostic in case of adenovirus 1 infection (canine viral hepatitis).

In canine laryngotracheitis mortality is very low. Intranuclear inclusion bodies are also seen in the epithelium of trachea.

Prevention and Treatment

Prevention is possible by vaccines given under the chapter on Distemper.

Other lines of treatment are symptomatic and hepatoprotective. Some drugs suggested for treatment are given below. Mortality is low.

Vaccines
1. Canigen DHPPi/L (Virbac) 5 vaccines in one
2. Canigen DHP vaccine against distemper, parvo, and adenovirus
3. Megavac 6: like canigen DHP (Indian Immunologicals Vaccine) + *Lepto canicola* and *L. icterohaemorrhagiae*
   Vaccination schedule: 1 ml by SC or IM route at 2, 3, 4 months and annually.
4. Duramune Max (Pfizer vaccine), like DHP
5. Venguard Plus 5 CVL (Pfizer vaccine)
6. Venguard 5 L: (Pfizer)

1. *Antibiotic injection:* To control secondary bacterial complications (Intaceph).
2. *Megludyne injection (Virbac):* Contains flunixin meglumine. Dose is 1 mg/kg/BW by slow IV or IM injection. This is to relieve pain, fever and swelling. (Flunimeg of Zydus can be used as alternative).

3. *Kepoliv solution:* To protect the liver by herbal combination, for general weakness. Dose: 5–7 ml daily (Kepler product).
4. *Belamyl iMnjection:* Contains thiamine, riboflavin niacinamide and B_{12} to treat anorexia. Dogs/cats: 0.5 to 1 ml IM injection daily.
5. *Liverolin (pet liver tonic with Silymarin):* A herbal product (Pfizer, packing of 150 ml). Dose: 1/2 teaspoon 2–3 times or for larger breed 5 ml 2–3 times a day.

   Other liver tonics are:
   - Livoferol (Cargil), liquid
   - Gutwell (Venky's Pet): 2 g to 5 g/day depending on the size of dog
   - Yakrifit (Ayurvet): Herbal
   - Hitone (Lyka)
   - Cholymbi (Lyka): Choline containing hepatoprotective
   - Liv 52 (Himalaya): Drops
   - Liv-T of SBL (Homoeopathic): 2 teaspoonful, 3–4 times daily

   Homoeopathic: Livtone (JVS Pharma): liquid tonic; 110, 200, and 500 ml; Dose: 2 teaspoons 3 times a day.

▓ CORONAVIRUS INFECTIONS (DOGS)

Canine coronavirus infection (CCV) is a highly contagious intestinal disease all over the world. The virus multiplies in the epithelium of small intestine. It produces a mild disease with slight or no symptoms but in combined infection with canine parvovirus or other intestinal pathogens, the disease becomes severe.

Symptoms

Vomiting and a few days of explosive diarrhoea (liquid, yellow-green or orange coloured).

Fever is very rare. Sometimes, mild respiratory problem and dehydration are observed in young dogs. In puppies, severe enteritis may cause death.

Infection

Exposure to feaces from infected dog. The virus persists up to six months post-infection. Overcrowding and unhygienic conditions help in the spread of the disease.

Diagnosis

Specific diagnosis is difficult but serological tests are practically difficult.

▓ FELINE ENTERIC CORONAVIRUS INFECTION IN CATS

It is a somewhat similar disease as of dogs.

▓ CORONAVIRUS DISEASE IN CALVES

Pathogenesis of coronavirus disease in calves is similar to rotavirus infection. In fact, viral diarrhoea in calves is caused by rotavirus, coronavirus, toroviruses, and parvovirus.

Outbreak of diarrhoea is seen in 4 to 14 days age and sometimes up to 4 weeks age. Signs are profuse diarrhoea, slight fever and dehydration.

Treatment:
1. Oral and parenteral fluid and electrolyte therapy (Intalyte of Intas or Rintose (Vetoguind) are better.

2. Use of biochemic mixture of 9 medicines in clean water, preferably in warm water will promptly control diarrhoea, if given every 15 to 30 minutes.

Homoeopathic: 'Croton' 6 or 30 liquid given in water as drops will support biochemic therapy mentioned avove (please see under calf diseases).
This therapy is successful in all species as also in human beings.

Vaccines: Prevention in dogs is possible by multiple antigenic vaccines for dogs which may also include coronavirus antigen.

Example:
1. Vanguard Plus 5 CVL vaccine of Pfizer
2. Vanguard CV vaccine which is a specific coronavirus vaccine. The vaccine is given in dogs above 6 weeks age and three doses are repeated at weekly intervals. Then the dose is repeated annually.
3. Duramune Max 5CVK/4L vaccine of Pfizer contains antigens including coronavirus.

■ PARVOVIRUS INFECTION

Parvovirus produces serious disease in dogs. In dogs two forms of disease are seen.
1. *Cardiac form:* This form is seen in 2 to 8 week old puppies causing sudden death. Intranuclear inclusion bodies are seen in heart muscles.
2. *Intestinal form:* Intestinal parvovirus infection occurs in all age groups but more severely in dogs older than 6 weeks.

Symptoms

Main symptoms are vomiting, diarrhoea (mostly bloody), fever, and leucopenia. The virus is 98% identical to feline panleukopenia, hence it also causes necrotising enteritis.

Treatment

1. Prevention is best for dogs for which multicomponent vaccines with distemper are already mentioned.
2. Intravenous drips with Ringers lactate solution (50 ml/kg) having electrolytes is given intravenously twice a day to stop dehydration.
3. Aciloc injection (2 ml/kg) can be mixed in Ringers lactose fluid for IV injection (slow).
4. Metronidazole liquid 20 mg/kg can also be mixed in Ringers lactose injection (injectable metronidazole).
   The dog may get cured after 3 to 15 days of treatment.
5. *Homoeopathic:* I had a wonderful success by treatment of a hopeless case of bloody diarrhoea and bloody moviting by homoeopathic medicine in a case of Parvo in terminal stage. Haemoglobin was 5 g/dl.
   I used: a. Phosphorus 200 2 to 3 drops in a little water by mouth, repeated every 15–20 minutes. With improvement, the interval was prolonged. Croton 6 or 30 was similarly given in water a few minutes before or after phosphorus. The result was impressive, which stopped the symptoms in less than 1 hour and the dog recovered and terurned to normal. Treatment for anaemia (Ferritas injection and Sharkoferal orally) was continued for several weeks.

■ FELINE PANLEUKOPENIA

(Agranulocytosis, Feline Distemper, Feline enteritis)

Hosts: Cats, cheetah, leopard, tiger

Etiology: Parvovirus. Infection spreads by direct contact. Virus is present in all secretions and faeces for ½ (1 and half) months post infection.

Signs: Diphasic fever for about 24 hours, subsides for next 24 hours and rises again after 48 hours. Temperature goes up to 104–105°F. Most important clinical finding is leucopenia with agranulocytosis. Intranuclear eosinophilic inclusion bodies in intestinal epithelium of eroded intestinal mucosa are seen microscopically. Cardiac form is also seen.

Fel-O-Vax Vaccine

Indications: Protection against panleukopenia, feline rhinocracheitis and calci virus.

Dosage: Vaccinate healthy cats 8 weeks of age or older with one 1 ml dose, followed by a second 1 ml dose three to four weeks later IM or SC. Cats vaccinated at less than 12 weeks of age should be given an additional 1 ml dose of vaccine at 12 to 16 weeks of age. Annual revaccination with a single dose of vaccine is recommended.

Feligen CRP vaccine: It is a triple vaccine. It contains:
  i. Feline panleucopenia vaccine
 ii. Feline viral rhincotracheitis vaccine
iii. Feline calcivirus vaccine

Vaccine: It is a freeze dreid vaccine. Dilute the vaccine with diluents provided with the vial.

Dose: Inject 1 ml vaccine SC irrespective of age, breed or weight of the animal.

Presentation: 1 ml × 10 vials with 10 diluents

■ FELINE CALCIVIRUS DISEASE

This disease is characterised by formation of vesicles in the nostrils, tongue and mouth which turn into sharply demarcated ulcers. Enteritis and arthritis are also observed. Acute respiratory disease and fever are first detected.

■ FELINE VIRAL RHINOTRACHEITIS

This is a disease of young recently weaned kittens. There is some fever and copious nasal discharge. In older cats mild nasal discharge is seen. The epithelium of mouth, larynx and trachea get necrosed which then ulcerate. Intranuclear inclusion bodies are found in the affected epithelium or trachea or nose.

Treatment: Rhus Tox 1000: 1 drop in water three times a day and Argentum nitricum 1000 2 drops in morning may be tried.

■ PAPILLOMA VIRUS INFECTIONS IN DOGS

The disease is called canine oral (mouth) papilloma of dogs.

Other diseases are:
 • *Cattle:* Skin papilloma (bovine type 1 and type 3)
 • *Cattle:* Teat papilloma (bovine type 5 and 6)

- *Horse:* Equine sarcoid, skin granuloma caused by bovine type 1)
- *Horse:* Equine papilloma virus; skin papilloma
  Ovine and caprine papilloma virus
  Fibropapilloma is rough cauliflower like growth, seen sometimes in cattle.
  In all these diseases the causes are papilloma viruses.
  There is no commercial vaccine for papilloma. I have used the following homoeopathic medicines with success:

1. *Thuza 1000:* In cattle, 15–20 drops by mouth (every 3–4 days) and application of Thuza Q externally daily.
2. *Wartoline drops:* 10 to 20 drops in some water in small animals and calves. The same medicine can be applied on warts 3 times daily (without water)(J.V.S. Pharma, Wazirpur Industrial area, N. Delhi) e-mail: jvspharma@yahoo.co.in
3. *Autogenous vaccine:* Wart tissue is homogenized in 50% glycerine saline (30 ml per gm of tissue) filter through muslin cloth, add dicrysticine 0.5 ml per 100 ml trichurate and 0.4 ml formalin per 100 ml. Keep at 4 °C for 24 hours. Inject 15 ml of this vaccine at the rate of 15 ml SC, twice a week. (Inayat et al 1999. Pakistan Vet. J. 19: 102).

▇ CANINE INFLUENZA (DOG FLU)

The disease is caused by various influenza viruses A such as equine influenza virus (H3 N8) and H3N2, a mutant of avian influenza virus. There is no evidence of transfer to people, cats, etc.

Symptoms

About 80% dogs have mild and 20% have subclinical disease and death is less than 1%. If the dog is protected with kennel cough vaccine then the possibility of influenza is less. Watery or greenish discharge, slight fever are observed. If untreated, up to 50% may develop pneumonia.

Treatment

1. *Allergia (Vetina Product):* Contains Quercetin (natural Benadryl), antioxidant, anti-inflammatory antiallergic components and vitamins A, C, E, green tea, etc.
   - *Packing:* 1 × 30 tablets.
   - *Dose:* Orally, mix with food.
   - *Up to 5 kg:* 1/2 tablet twice a day.
   - *Up to 10 kg:* 1 tablet twice daily.
2. *Vet DMG:* (*Vetina Product*).
   Syrup: 30 ml; dose: 0.25 ml per 5 kg BW twice a day; 2 ml 35–45 kg BW twice a day.
3. *Kemolide (Kepler Product):* Nimesulide 100 mg: dogs 2–3 ml injection twice a day.
   Paracetamol —150 mg if there is fever.
   Dose: Pets—2 to 3 ml orally.
4. Marbomet tablets (Nuvo/Intas) —Marbofloxacin.
   Give 2–5 mg per kg BW orally once a day for 3 to 5 days.
5. *Kepflu injection:* In serious cases, 0.5 ml/10 kg BW, daily.
6. *Antibiotics:* If there is fever, give antibiotic injections as listed in index of drugs.

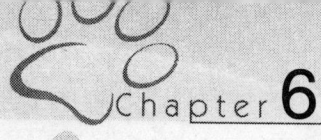

Chapter 6

Wounds and Pain

Wounds are the commonest problem in all the animals of all species including pets. Causes are very variable but mostly they are due to physical injury or accident.

STEP I: TREATMENT

Ordinary wounds may be treated by any of the dozens of antiseptic ointments available in the market. The wounds should be washed and cleaned with antiseptic lotion, dilute alcohol or iodine. Then apply ointments such as Betadine liquid.

1. *Negasunt (Bayer)* 100 ml liquid: Spray on the wound area twice daily. This can also be used for wounds of feet, FMD, surgical wounds, naval infections. Negasunt powder is also applied twice daily (all animals including dogs).

2. *Topicure (ointments and spray):* This is a herbal product of Natural Remedies which is antiseptic and anti-inflammatory. It is used as spray even for inflamed udder, feet, etc. The animal may not allow any other application due to pain hence spray is good. 'Scavon' spray of Himalya Drugs is similar to Topicure.

   Kiskin cream and lotion (Intas Pharma) are very good for ringworm, allergic dermatitis, eczema, fungal infections, cuts, wounds, pyoderma, surgical wounds, and burns.

3. Parenteral injections of antibiotics may be required in case of complicated, deep-seated, infected wounds, e.g. *Bayrocin:* This is available as 100 ml of 10% Enrofloxacin which is a broad-spectrum antibiotic.

   Dose: 2.5–5 ml per 100 kg BW daily for 3–5 days as IM, IV or SC route.

   Bayrocin 1 shot: Contains 100 mg/ml. Bayrocin can be used in all cloven footed animals. This is given by SC route and acts for 48 hours it is repeated after 48 hours. Dose 7.5–12.5 ml/100 kg BW (30 and 50 ml vial).

   Ampillin injection of Lyca, Baxivet (ampicillin + dicloxacillin) of Lyca, Lykacef vet injection (It is a new generation antibiotic for serious cases). Dose of Lykaceft injection is 5–10 mg/kg BW or even 15 mg to 25 mg/kg BW in dogs and cats by IM or IV route. *Megadox-N of Neospark* is available as 50 g pack of doxycylin and *neomycin* of Neospark Co which is given orally at the rate of 10–20 mg per kg BW for 3–5 days. *Duxprim* of neospark contains trimethoprim and sulphamethoxazole. It is given orally at the rate of 2.5 g per 10 kg BW. *Enrostrong* (Enrofloxacin) is an oral solution to be given at the rate of 0.5 to 1 ml/10 kg BW for 3–5 days. *Enrostrong (PZ) injection of Mankind* Co is to be given as a single vial in large animals daily for 3–5 days. It also contains Pefloxacin. *Serakind Plus* is a bolus of Mankind to reduce swelling around the wound or yoke gall. It contains seraptopeptidase paracetamol and meloxicam. Dose: 2 bolus daily in large and 1 bolus in small animals.

■ STEP II: NUTRITIONAL SUPPLEMENTS

Give vitamin C orally or as *ascorbic acid injection* (5 ml, Juggat) on alternate days. Cecon tablets. Tota Vit Strong (mixture) of Mankind is available in banana flavor for dogs. It contains methochelated 5 vitamins, 12 minerals, 2 amino acids and 2 probiotics for fast recovery. For large animals *Tota Vit Strong* of Mankind can be given at the rate of 30–50 g mixture daily by oral route.

Glosacc AV (Intas) is a liquid nutritional supplement having amino acids, minerals, plant extracts, and vitamins. Packing of 1L bottle.

Dose: 1 ml/litre in drinking water.

RBC RAKKT: Multimineral, and vitamin containing oral tonic for anaemia in liquid form. Dose: Cattle: 40–50 ml daily goat, sheep, calves: 10–15 ml.

Packing is of 500 ml.

■ STEP III: ANTITETANUS INJECTION

Should never be forgotten for valuable animals and manufactured also by Dano Vaccine and Biologicals as 5 ml ampoule. It is given at the rate of 0.5 ml as deep intramuscular injection one shot.

■ STEP IV: ANAEMIA + WOUND

If there is too much bleeding and if haemoglobin drops below 8 g/dl then give iron tonic like Sharkoferd syrup of Alembic orally. Or injections of Ferritas (Intas). Inject 1 ml/50 kg BW 10 ml vial). 1 bolus (strips of 5 boli); 2 boli/day/orally for adult and 1/2 bolus for small animals for 14 days.

Liver supplements: Hepotas (Intas Pharma), Liv 52

Belamyl injection, Livoforol, Livotas, etc. may be given orally or as injections if needed. *Kepatite of Kepler Co is bolus for cattle* which improves appetite and provides minerals.

■ STEP V: SHOCK AND FLUID BALANCE

Inerol (Intas) contains isoflupredone. It is given as injection to save from shock, inflammation, myositis, arthritis, tenosynovitis, and ketosis. (5 and 10 ml containing risoflupredone; inject 5–10 ml in large animals and 2.5 to 5 ml in calves at the rate of 1 ml per 50 kg BW by IM route, or IV route in urgency; per day or twice a day (slow)

Prednisoleng injection (MSD product): 0.5 mg per kg BW; 5–10 ml for cattle by SC route.

■ STEP VI: PAIN

To take care of pain
1. *Vetalgin vet* (MSD injection)—Contains Analgin 50%. It treats any type of pain including wounds, gastric pain, reproductive pain, etc. Packing of 33 ml.
   Dose: IV or IM injection, cattle 20–40 ml; horse 40–60 ml, calf 5–15 ml; sheep/goat 2–8 ml; dog 1–5 ml.
2. *Maxxtol -XP* (Telfenamic acid 60 mg/ml injection)
   20 ml vial: Dose: IM or IV injection at the rate of 4 mg/kg (0.5 ml) as a single dose and half the dose for repeating after 48 hours.

3. *Melonex of Intas* or *Melobest of TTK Healthcare, Melambic injection of Alembic* and *Melambic P (Paracetamol)*
   a. *Meloxicam 5 mg/ml:* Inject for pain due to any disease in the body and before and after surgery.
      Dose: Dog—0.2 to 0.5 ml/10 kg BW.
             Cattle—30 ml/300 kg BW (Packing of 2, 15, 30, and 100 ml).
   b. *Melonex bolus:* (100 mg × 4 boli) *Melambic P bolus of Alembic* and *Melobest P bolus* of TTK.
      Large animal—2 boli/400 kg BW orally, daily.
      Small animal—1/4 to 1/2 bolus daily.
   c. *Melonex Plus:* Paracetamol and lignocaine with meloxicam.
      Inject 30 ml/400 kg BW or 1 ml/10 kg BW; dog 0.2 to 0.5 ml (packing of 30 and 100 ml vial).
   d. *Melonex XZ Plus* (Intas injection containing paracetamol and serraoto peptidase with meloxicam, 4 boli × 10 strips).
      Serratiopeptidase removes exudate (swelling) in inflamed area by removing proteins of exudates.
      Dose: 1 bolus/250 kg BW daily, orally.
   e. *Melonex (Power) injection (meloxicam + lignocaine; 20 mg and 1%).*
   f. *Melonex plus bolus (100 mg + 1500 mg paracetamol).*
4. *Ketonit* (Ketoprophen injection 100 mg) for pain in joints, muscles, colic, wounds, and fever.
   Packing injections: 15 and 90 ml vials of Tineta Pharma.
   Dose: 12–15 ml, IV/IM injection for large animals.
5. *Xylazine injection* (G. Loucatos Co., Mumbai)—diclofenac sodium with paracetamol injection.
   A sedative, anaesthetic and muscle relaxant. Packing of 2, 10 and 30 ml vial.
6. *Nimesulide containing drugs* such as Rely NP of Lyka. Bolus of 4 × 1 strip. Large animals 1–2 bolus twice a day; small animals 1/2 bolus.
7. *Spasmovet injection* of Vetoquinol: Contains Dicyclomine. Relieves both spasms and pain. Dose 1 ml/20 kg BW; dog 0.5–2 ml, IM injection, 12 hourly.
8. *Vetoprofen* (Merial Co. Product): Contains 100 mg ketoprofen per ml. Dose, etc. as for ketonil.
9. *Ketop of Alembic* (same as Vetprofem).
10. *Aletol of Alembic:* Injection of Tolfenamic (30 and 100 ml) treats pain, inflammation and fever. Dose: 40 mg per 10 kg (1 ml) BW.

■ STEP VII: MAGGOTED WOUNDS

To stop maggots in wounds or to remove them from wound, some special treatment is needed. For example:
1. *Dospray (Merial product):* Antiseptic maggoticidal fly repellent spray. It contains Hexachloride protavine (1%), hemisulfate (0.1%), etrimide (0.45%). It can also be used to treat lesions of FMD, Degnala disease and foot rot.
   Sprayed 2–3 times a day (100 ml tin).
2. *Safroid spray of Kepler Co. (75 ml):* It is an ayurvedic drug for deep wounds, maggoted wounds, septic, fungal infections, etc.

3. *Dermichlor spray*: Product of Vetoquinol Co, Mumbai. Treats skin infections of Staphylococci, Malassezia, *Microsporum canis*, *M. gypsum* and Trichophyton in dogs (Antifungal)
   Use: Bathe, groom or shake and spray bottle (100 ml).
   Spray (sparing eyes, nose and mouth) from a distance of 15 cm, opposite to the direction of hair. Air dry skin and repeat next day.
4. *Lorexane cream* and spray by Virbac: Fly repellent, healing of open wounds.

STEP VIII: HOMOEOPATHIC DRUGS FOR WOUNDS, SPRAINS, AND INFLAMMATION

Calendula ointment: Calendula ointment is one of the best for shortest healing and antisepsis.

Calendula 30 globules: Give 5–6 globules to dogs or cats and 10–15 drops in water to cattle, buffaloes, sheep, goats and dogs 3 times a day.

Hepar Sulph and Silicia 200: Give 5–6 drops TDS if there is pus in wound. It is extremely good.

STEP IX: DEBILITY IN INJURED ANIMALS

1. *Toldim Phos injection:* (Tineta Product)
2. Five phos tablets (homoeopathic) 5 tablets TDS in small animals.

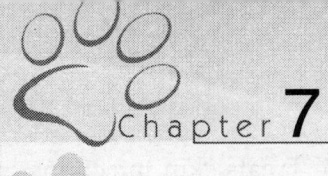

Chapter 7

Miscellaneous Diseases

■ HYPOTHYROIDISM

In dogs, 95% cases of hypothyroidism are due to autoimmune damage in the form of atrophic thyroiditis. T_4 harmone is deiodinated to T_3. T_4 (thyroxin) is bound to plasma proteins (99%)/Free T_4 (f T_4) is active form which also controls TSH secretion by pituitary. T_3 is biologically inactive product of T_4.

Susceptible breeds: Hypothyroidism is seen in only 0.2% of the dog population. Most of the recognised breeds are susceptible.

Signs

1. Peripheral neuropathies (facial nerve paralysis, forelimb lameness
2. Bilaterally symmetrical alopecia
3. Recurrent pyoderma
4. Hyperpigmentation and scale formation
5. Obesity and lethargy
6. Bradycardia (increased heartbeat)
7. Weakness
8. Lipid deposits in cornea.

Clinical Diagnosis

ECG

1. Bradycardia, low voltages in all leads and inversion of T wave
2. Unresponsive anaemia in 20–32% dogs
3. Higher ESR
4. Hypercholesterolemia (70% of cases)
5. Hyperlipidemia (lipid profile)

T_4 test

It is good test and nonexpensive. In 89 out of 100 it is low.

Antibody test for lymphocytic thyroiditis: Around 50% dogs show positive anti-thyroglobulin antibodies due to leakage of thyroglobulin (ELISA test) out of gland.

Treatment

Thyroxine supplementation in the dose of 30 mg/kg should be started (12 hourly doses).

Lethargy, etc. show improvement in about 3 weeks.

T_4 concentration should rise to 2.0 to 4.5 mg/dl with progress (25 to 60 mmol/dl).

Normal values: T_3 —1.15 to 3.16 nmol/: or 0.154 µg/dl
T_4—0.078 µg/dl
TSH—0.00 to 0.35 ng/ml

Treatment

When T_4 supplementation fails then synthetic triiodothyronine is indicated.

▨ EPILEPSY IN DOGS

About 25 to 50% of epilepsy cases are not satisfactorily controlled. Epilepsy in dogs are of two types:
1. Primary or true or idiopathic which is possibly due to genetic inheritance.
2. Symptomatic or acquired:—This is due to intracranial or extracranial disease (tumours, inflammation, trauma, etc). Hence, history is to be taken carefully.

History

In primary or idiopathic type, first seizure occurs between 1 to 5 years age. If the disease is seen below or above this age then a causal disease can be investigated.
It can also be a. generalised.

Localized

Generalised: Opisthotonos or paddling with or without salivation, urination or defecation.
In localized form, tail chasing, fly biting, twitching of some parts of body are observed.

Laboratory Tests

a. Cerebrospinal fluid examination: To know inflammatory condition in CNS.
b. Liver function test (to rule out hepatic encephalopathy).
c. Rule out ketamine or ivermectin treatment or change in dog's routine or environment.

Antiepileptic Drugs

1. Phenobarbital—dose 2 to 5 mg/kg twice a day for 10 to 18 days.
2. Valproate: 60 mg/kg 3 times a day.
3. Mephentoin: 10 mg/kg 3 times a day for 5 to 7 days.
4. Potassium bromide—20 mg/kg once a day for 4 months.
Combined therapy of phenobarbital and potassium bromide may bring about polyuria, polydipsia, polyphagia and sedation.

Status Epilepticus

Diazepam, 10–35 mg in bolus form may give temporary relief for other steps to follow. In case of status epilepticus, 50% dextrose/IV may also be injected because hypoglycaemia is often seen in status epilepticus. Calcium may also be injected if hypocalcaemia is also seen. Gardenal tablets of Piramal Health Care (phenobarbital sodium) available as 10, 20, 30, and 60 mg tablets can be given for long-term management. It is to be given orally in food at the rate of 2–5 mg per kg twice a day.

If the dog remains seizure-free for 1 or 2 years then the treatment may be withdrawn gradually. Steady period of seizures at 3–4 months gap indicates good progress. Seizures of less than 1 per week frequency need maintenance.

■ DERMATITIS (DOGS)

Dermatitis is very common in dogs, usually with erythema, hyperpigmentation or diffuse alopecia.

Causes

1. Parasites—ticks, lice infestation
2. Bacterial—with slight fever
3. Allergic—with itchig and pruritus

Treatment

Antihistaminic: Antihistaminic ointments such as 'Surfaz' cream which contains antibacterial antiallergic and antifungal components.

Wokazole Plus (30 and 100 ml *liquid*): Apply lotion twice a day. Treats fungal, bacterial infections, dermatitis and alopecia.

Ketochlor shampoo—(antifungal and antibacterial)
   If there are nodular (urticarial) and pyodermatitis then apply 'Wakazole lotion'. Then any one antibiotic injection (generally, clindamycin 10 mg/kg BW by IM for 1 to 3 days. After 1 week, only topical lotion or shampoo is continued
   Spectrazole (Pfizer) liquid 2, 30, 100, ml treats bacterial, fungal infection and eczema. Apply 2–3 times a day.

If allergic (generalized)

1. *Prednisolone injection* 0.25 to 0.5 mg per kg as IM injections or Curadex injection 2 ml IM/day (Concept).
2. *Chlorpheneramin maleate injection* in above dose and route
   Or *'Sheen an Clean'* shampoo of Venkeys is effective for bacterial and fungal dermatitis.
   Enrofloxacin 1 mg/kg/IM for 7 days with antihistaminics given above for treatment of bacterial dermatitis.

Nutritional Dermatitis

Synoderm: A product of Veteran Laboratory, Bengaluru which contains zinc, sulphur and cobalt is given at the dose rate of 1 tablet BID for 7 days. Synoderm treatment results in recovery, mosty in 7 days. Treatment with antibiotics and antihistamine drugs takes about 2 weeks.

Parasitic Dermatitis

Scrotal Dermatitis: Scrotum becomes red and moist. Treatment with ampicillin and cloxacillin injection at the dose rate of 10 mg/kg by IM route twice a day is given till recovery. 'Topicure' spray of natural remedies twice a day helps in recovery. *Dermocept* cream (Concept), a herbal antiallergic, antifungal, antieczema, also cures mange and wounds.

Demodicotic Dermatitis: In this disease there is alopecia, papules, scaling, crusting and hyperpigmentation all over the body. Demodex canis mites can be seen in large numbers in skin scrapings (up to 40 or so/per field).

Treatment: Inject ivermectin with complete cure by 6th week with improvement by 2nd week. Complete recovery is confirmed till 2 skin scrapings are negative. Bright hair coat starts by 7th week.

Lusfur liquid, a product of Kepler (Ahmedabad; phone 079-30144400) contains neem, coconut, heena, and alovera. This fluid is applied to affected skin at the rate of 7 to 10 ml. It is rubbed for 5–10 minutes.

Petsyl: Tablets containing 2 mg ivermectin and praziquintel 50 mg per tablet is given at the dose of 1 tablet per 10 kg BW once a week. This tablet kills all ectoparasites, hookworms, roundworms, whipworms, lungworms, tapeworms, tick, mites, lice, fleas, etc.

Ceftiforce (Mankind): Ceftriaxone, inject 10 mg/kg BW, IM or IV for 3–5 days for bacterial infections.

Seborrhoeic dermatitis: use 'Micodin' shampoo (Intas). Allow to act for 5–10 minutes, then wash. Repeat 2–3 times a week.

Recurrent Demedecosis: Give oral ivermectin 300 mg/kg/day and cefotaxime sodium 20 mg/kg BW twice a day. Examine the skin scrapping weekly till hairs appear (generally after 3 weeks). Repeat weekly for another 2 weeks. Use 'Kiskin ' ointment (Intas) 3–4 times a day.

■ LARGE AREA SKIN LOSS AND INFECTED WOUND

Generally due to accidents, a large wound devoid of skin may come for treatment. Plastic surgery is the proper treatment but this is not possible by all practitioners. The steps to be taken are:

1. Remove mud, sand, etc. by antiseptic washing such as by 'Dettol' antiseptic wash or Betadine liquid.
2. Clean with normal saline and apply povidone iodine ointment and dress with Robert Jones bandage.
3. Repeat dressing on alternate days for 10 days.
4. Apply 'Calendula' homoeopathic ointment from 2nd day
5. Give Calendula 30 globules (6–8) orally before meals 2–3 times a day.
6. Recovery takes maximum of 10 weeks
7. Newcharm: Skin gel of Ayurvet helps in cure of ringworm, pyoderma and demodicosis. For external use or Healokind spray (Mankind) daily till recovey.

■ PYOMETRA (ACCUMULATION OF PUS IN UTERUS)

Renukaradhya, GG et al, 2010, National Congress on Canine Practice, Jan 21-23, 2010)—*for dogs:*

1. Treat with 10 mg/kg/day with Miphistone orally for 3 days.
2. SC injection of 10 mg/kg of PGF_2 (carboprost tromethamine) twice a day for 3 days.
3. Ampicillin cloxacillin injection twice a day for 3 weeks.
   Leucocytosis above 30,000 may come down to normal.
   Injection of prostaglandin (PGF_2) caused retching, vomiting, and abdominal straining within about 30 minutes.

Cattle: Ceftatime (Mankind) injection containing Ceftiofur is injected IM, 24 hourly (1 g vial in 20 ml water) at the rate of 1.1 –2.2 mg/kg BW.

Small and medium breeds of dogs are more affected by pyometra (92/125) than large breeds (33/125). Age of the problem was more in more than 7 years old bitches (51%), about 40% in 4–6 years old bitches.

INDUCTION OF OESTRUM IN BITCHES

If bitches fail to exhibit oestrum for 8 to 10 months, it is due to hormonal imbalance including pseudopregnancy.

Cabergoline at the rate of 5 mcg/kg BW is given per os daily for 7 days and if needed, up to 10 days. Carbergoline is a long-acting dopamine which antagonizes prolacta. This is a safer drug than hormonal therapy. *Vitacept* (Concept) at the rate of 1–2 ml may also be injected at 5–6 days interval.

INFERTILITY IN BITCHES

Gyaecare', a nutritional supplement may be fed at the rate of 10 g per day for 10 days. This drug is reported to induce 77% conception after about 1 month (Chandrashekarmurty, A. et al 2010, coc cit).

OTITIS IN DOGS

Symptoms

Shaking of head, pruritis, discharge from ear and occasionally, drooping of ear.

Treatment

1. Clean aseptically the external ear on 3rd, 7th, 10th and 14th day.
2. Administer broad-spectrum antibiotic (cefimime) orally for 5 days. Enrocin (enrofloxacin) can be fed at the rate of 5 mg/kg BW for 3 to 5 days (Pfizer).
3. 'Cefovecin' (Pfizer) can be injected at the rate of 20 mg/kg BW once a day by IM route.
4. 'Otirel' eardrops (Pfizer) or 'Earwell' eardrops which have antibacterial, antifungal, antiallergic and anti-inflammatory action are good. Give till full recovery.
5. Gentamycin eardrops 3 times a day for 3 to 5 days after cleaning with ear bud.
   i. *In resistant cases:* Give ciprofloxacin or cephalexin or norfloxacin injection also.
   ii. Tab Flagyl or metronidazole 400 mg 2 times a day for 7 weeks.

TICS, LICE, MITES, AND FLEAS INFESTATION IN DOGS

Drugs for use:
1. 'Cisaflux' (Pfizer): Wet the dog hairs, apply shampoo, and massage into the body coat. Leave for some time. Rinse with water. Repeat once or twice a month for a few months.
2. 'Clavotin' —for mites and mange.
3. *Asuntal (soap by Bayer)*: Allow to act for 4–5 minutes then wash.

Generalised demodicosis, scabies and ear mites can be cured by ivermectin injection of any company including Clavotin. Dose is 0.2 to 0.5 mg per kg BW. *Clavotin* is available as 10 ml of 1% solution. This injection will be used for 20 kg dog or as 2 repeated injections.

Diptraz 12.5 (Merial): 15 and 50 ml pack. Apply on skin 1 ml/2 kg BW for ticks, lice. 3–4 ml for sarcoptic mange (2–3 applications). Demodectic mange 5–8 applications.

Kiltix collar: *It is a collar of Bayer* which is stretched 2–3 time and hung loosely on neck. It kills ticks and fleas (size medium and large).

◼ PYOMETRA AND METRITIS

Lixen IU: Lixen IU is ideal for endometritis and pyometra (Virback Animal Health). Lixen suspension contains 4 g cephalexin which makes 60 ml when reconstituted. The prepared infusion is infused into the uterus with AI gun.

Indications: Metritis, endometritis, cervicitis, pyometra and postpartum septic metritis.

Utro Met Bolus (Neospark): These boli contain nitrofurazone 60 mg and urea 6.0 g. 2 to 4 boli are introduced (in cows) into each horn of uterus after treating retained placenta. This prevents metritis, pyometra, etc.

Saftifur (Merial): Ceftifur sodium is presented as 1 g vial with 20 ml sterile water. The dissolved powder is injected at the dose rate 1.1 to 2.2 mg/kg BW as IM or SC injection daily for 3 to 5 days. It is useful for endometritis, pyometra, RDP besides foot rot, septicaemia, pneumonia, etc.

Uteriguard (Zydus): It contains cephalexin. It is to be used like lixen mentioned above.

Metricare IU (Zydus): It is available as 30 and 100 ml povidone iodine (50%) and metronidazole (1%). It stops repeat breeding of infectious origin, metritis, pyometra and eliminates all uterine infections and also helps reduce uterine prolapse. Administer 30–60 ml fluid by intrauterine route, twice at interval of 24 hours.

Furea U and *Furea U Plus:* Furea U Plus contains oxytetracyclin also. Presentation strip of 6 boli.

Use: As for metricare

Introduce 2 to 4 boli in each horn. Repeat after 24 hours. It also helps treat ROP, repeat breeding besides metritis and endometritis.

Oriprim U bolus (Zydus): Bolus contains trimethoprim sulphamethoxazole and urea. It is nontoxic nonirritant. Urea has proteolytic action hence helps the drugs to penetrate deep into the exudates.

Indications: ROP, enteritis, endometritis, pyometra repeat breeders.

Method: Place 2–4 boli into the uterus after parturition. Also dissolve 2 bol in sterile water and infuse into the uterus with AI pipette. This may be repeated next day.

Ergometrin (Zydus, injection of 5 ml): It is better to inject 2–5 mg/cow, buffalo, mare and 1/4th dose in sheep and goats by IV or IM injection to expel all exudates, placenta and also to help in involution of uterus. It also optimises intercalving interval.

◼ TICKS AND FLEAS IN DOGS

Fipronil (Sava Vet product) liquid 1 ml or more is to be poured at the middle of the back (pour on). The drug is available as per the weight of dog (up to 10 kg, 10–20 kg,

20–40 kg, 40–60 kg). After pouring, leave the dog without bathing. After 4th day, bathe the dog with antitick shampoo. The effect lasts for 1 month. *Cisa-Tix*: This is for 'Nonstop protection' against ticks, fleas, and lice in dogs and cats. It is available as 75 g container. Dust the body against the direction of hair and stroke the fur to rub the powder gently into the skin. Apply to feet, legs, and tail also but save the eyes and nose. Repeat once or twice every week or for extended period in heavy infestation. It contains 'Propoxur' 10 mg per gram of powder.

Cisa Flus: Instant treatment of ticks and fleas. Apply shampoo in wet hair. Leave for some time and wash. Do not use for cats.

Pro Meris Duo (Pfizer): This contains Metaflumizon, 150 mg/ml and Amitraz 150/ml. It is available as pack of 3 pipettes. It is to be used as per weight of dogs as follows:

Weight of dog	Pipette size to be used	Volume ml
Less than 5 kg	Pro Meris Duo small dogs	0.67
5.1–10 kg	Pro Meris Duo medium dogs	1.33
10.1–25 kg	Pro Meris Duo spot-on for medium and large dogs	3.33
25.1–40.0 kg	Pro Meris Duo spot on for large dogs	5.33

Tikkil shampoo (Indian Immuno) 100 ml Cypereathrin

Freedom spray (Venkys Pet, 100 and 225 ml) for ticks and fleas contains fipronil 0.25%. Spray all over the body from 10–20 cm distance.

Fur Free spray (Venkys Pet) is an anti-tick wash with Cypermethrin 1% as shampoo; available in 100 and 200 ml packs.

NT Mite: Contains Amitraz 12.5% for generalised demodecosis, scabies, ticks and fleas. 3–4 ml is dissolved per litre water and applied to skin.

■ URINARY TRACT INFECTIONS

Generally, this is suspected when there is pyrexia of unknown origin. It recurs again and again. Seftifur sodium injection is the drug of choice (Xenel, and other brands). For dogs, 250 mg injections by SC for prolonged period of 5 to 14 days. Marbomet (Intas) with Morbofloxacin is very good for urinary tract infections (UTIs), strip of 5 tablets of 50 mg each. Dose: (oral) 2–5 mg/kg BW once a day till recovery.

■ BACTERIAL INFECTIONS OF SKIN, SOFT TISSUES AND UPPER OR LOWER RESPIRATORY TRACT

Amoxicillin trihydrate and potassim clavulanate (clavulanic acid) 200 mg and 28.5 mg respectively are available as oral suspension (Temobax by Pfizer). It is to be given at the rate of 12.5–25 mg/kg BW or 5 ml per 10 kg BW, orally for 3 to 5 days. Mix (for Trombax, Pfizer) in 30 ml water. Shake well and give orally.

■ WORMS IN DOGS

The important roundworms, tapeworms and Cestodes are listed below:

Toxocara canis (roundworms): Located in small intestine of dogs and fox. Symptoms include diarrhoea and anorexia.

Ancylostoma caninum: Hookworms are blood sucking worms which may cause anaemia and anorexia.

Spirocarcalupi: Roundworms in nodules formed in oesophagus. Symptoms: Dysphagia.

Dirofilaria immitis: It is called heartworm; located in right ventricle and right pulmonary artery.

Symptoms: Coughing, hypertrophy of right ventricle; passive venous congestion, liver enlargement and ascites. This is found all over India.

Diagnosis: A diagnostic kit called SNAP 4 DX Plus produced by IDEXX Laboratories B.V. P.O. Box1334 NL 2130, EK, Hootddarp, U.S.A. is available for field diagnosis like Brucella kit. Worms are 12 to 30 cm long (Recorded in Bihar and Gujarat).

Whipworms

Tapeworms: Dipylidium caninum: It is located in small intestine of dogs, cats, foxes. Occasionally, multiceps multiceps is found in the intestine of dogs.

All the above worms can be expelled or killed by broad-spectrum drugs. Examples are:

Plozin which contains fenbendazole, praziquintel and pyrantel. *Plozin plus* is for bigger dogs, in the form of tablets.

Dose: 'Plozin': 1 tablet per 10 kg BW. Repeat every 3 months (Pfizer product).

'Plozin Plus': 1 tablet per 25 kg BW; repeat 3 monthly.

'Catel' (Pfizer): Controls roundworms, tapeworms, hookworms and whipworms. It has the broadest spectrum. It also contains oxantel embonate besides praziquintel and pyrental embonate.

Dose: 1 tablet per 10 kg BW by mouth. Repeat 3 monthly

Prazital Forte (Indian Immunologicals): Acts against roundworms, hookworms, and tapeworms, including eggs and larvae. Packing of 20 × 2 tablets. Dose: 1 tablet per 10 kg BW.

Ivectin (ivermectin 10 mg tablets: Removes ecto and endoparasites including mange. Dose: Dog 6 mcg/kg/day for 1 month. Cat 24 mcg/day/month.

Neomac injection (Intas): Ivermectin 0.3 mg/kg BW, SC 1, 7, 10, 20, and 50 ml vials.

Chapter 8

Protozoal Blood Infections

BABESIOSIS

Babesiosis (red water fever, cattle tick fever, piroplasmosis): Babesia are tick borne intraerythrocytic parasites of veretebrates. Prevalent in tropical and subtropical countries.

Hosts	Causal agent (only important ones)	Ticks
Dogs	Babesia, Canis, *B. gibsoni*	Dog ticks
Cattle	Babesia bovis	Boophilus
Buffalo	*B. bigemina*	Boophilus
Sheep	*B. motasi*	Rhiphicephalus
Goats	*B. ovis*	Rhiphicephalus
Horse	*B. equi, B. caballi*	Dermacentor, etc.

Adult infected hosts may serve as carriers for as long as 2 years. Wild animals may act as reservoirs. Contaminated needle may transfer infection from animal to animal. Both humoral and cellular immunity are responsible for protection. Age related immunity also helps up to 6 months after birth of calf. Post Babesia infection immunity is also strong.

Pathogenesis

Most Babesia sporozoits enter into erythrocytes and cycle of asexual multiplication starts. Destruction of RBCs results in haemolysis, anaemia, jaundice, and haemoglobinuria. There is blood stasis, thrombosis in heart and brain in acute form.

In cattle the disease runs for 3 to 7 days with fever of 40°C or more. Haemoglobinuria (red water) is often present. Later, weakness and jaundice develop. In subacute form in younger animals fever is mild and haemoglobinuria is absent. Haemoglobinuria is more likely in B. bigemina infection.

Sheep: As in cattle.

Horses: Lateral recombancy, anorexia, fever and oedomatous swellings in fetlocks, sometimes colic jaundice is more often seen in young horses.

Diagnosis

Direct amination of blood smears stained with Giemsa or Leishmans stain. Blood from tip of tail or ears is more likely to show parasites. RBCs just below the fluffy coat are more likely to have parasites. Other tests include immunofluorescence, ELISA, etc.

Signs: Fever, more than 107°F, lymph nodes swelling, lacrimation, and nasal discharge, anorexia, anaemia with/without jaundice.

Buparvaquone 2.5 mg/kg BW by IM route is given as a single injection, e.g. 'Butalex' of Novartis, 'Berenil' of MSD can be given or 'Kepaquone' of Kepler for treatment.

Dimindzene Aceturate with Phenazone (Batrynil of Zydus) can treat babesiosis, trypanosomiasis and PUO (30 and 90 ml bottles are available).

Dose: 5–10 ml/100 kg BW by deep IM injection.

Deminacure injection (Bayer): Contains diminazine aceturate 70 mg and phenazone 375 mg per ml. It is used for babesiosis, trypanosomiasis and mixed hemoprotozoal diseases. Dose is 5 ml per 100 kg BW by deep IM route. Double dose is used in severe cases.

Differential Diagnosis of Haemoprotozoan Diseases

Symptoms	Babesiosis	Theileriosis	Trypanosomiasis	Anaplasmosis
Fever	Present	Present	Present	Present
Lymph nodes prescapular or femoral	Normal	Swollen	Normal	Normal
Haemoglobinuria	Present	Absent	Absent	Absent
Nervous signs	Absent	Absent	Present	Absent
Jaundice/Icterus	Occasionally present	Present	Absent	Occasionally present
Abortion	Occasionally occurs	Absent	Absent	Occasionally occurs
Nasal discharge	Absent	Present	Absent	Absent
Lacrimation	Absent	Present	Absent	Absent
Pin point haemorr-hages in conjunctiva	Absent	Present	Absent	Absent

Theileriasis is the most important haemoprotozoan disease. The above chart can help in clinical diagnosis and treatment. It is also most common cause of pyrexia of unknown origin (PUO).

As reported by NK Singh et al (Compendium, Indian Society for Advencement of Canine practice 7th Annual Convention, 21-23, 2010) 5 years of study revealed the following:

Dogs

- Total positive patients: 7.08% (55/776)
- Trypanosome evansi: 7.27%
- Babesiosis: 65.45%
- Ehrlichia canis: 21.80%
- Hepatozoon canis: 5.45%

Most prevalent was babesiosis. The best way in my view is to centrifuge the blood in haematocrit tube and then prepare smears from RBCs just below the buffy coat. Presence of pear or teardrop-shaped parasites in pairs or singles after Giemsa staining or Wrights Giemsa staining allows good and reliable diagnosis.

Treatment

1. *Batrynil* ve RTU injection (contains diminazine aceturate 20 mg and phenazone 375 mg) per ml.
   Use: Treats babesiosis, trypanosomiasis and also pyrexia of unknown origin (PUO).
2. *Nilbery*: Similar to Batrynil (Intas), available in 30 ml and 90 ml vials.
3. *Prozomin* (Virbac) similar to Batrynil.
4. *Trityl* (Lyca): Injection, same as for Batrynil (30 and 100 ml vials).
5. *Zokil* (Mankind): 30 ml injection.
6. *Lytrip* (Lyka): Injection or prevention and treatment of trypanosomiasis.
   Dose: 4.4 mg/kg BW, SC injection.
7. *Surral*: Alembic injection 0.5 mg/kg BW by deep IM injection.
8. *Nyzem*: For trypanosomiasis, deep IM injection of 1 mg/kg BW (pack of 250 mg vial).

▇ THEILERIASIS (EAST COAST FEVER; TURNING SICKNESS)

It is a tick born protozoan disease very common in India. There are several species. As a rare complication, brain may be involved resulting in 'Turning sickness'.

Etiology

Parasite	Int. host (ticks)	Host
Bab. bovis	Boophilus	Cattle
Theileria parva	Rhipicephalus appendiculatus; R. zambeziensis (brown eartick)	Cattle/buffalo. In India local breeds of cattle develop some resistance which may be broken by wet, hot, humid season
T. annulata	Hyalomma	Cattle, buffalo
T. mutans	Amblyomma sp.	Cattle, buffalo
T. ovis	Rhipicephalus sp. For all these parasites	*T. ovis* affects sheep
T. hirci		*T. hirci* affects goats
T. taurotragi	Rhipicephalus sp	Cattle, sheep

Clinical findings: The parasites are found in RBCs as round, coccobacillary, comma-shaped or ring-shaped bodies. In WBCs and monocytes they appear as multiple bunch of purple stained schizonts called 'Koch's blue bodies' when stained by Giemsa stain. In brain, these infected cells may block small capillaries with or without infarction, resulting in 'Turning sickness'. Panleukopenia and thrombocytopenia may also be observed.

Symptoms: Generalised enlargement of lymph nodes, emaciation, weakness, recumbancy, nasal and ocular discharge, swollen conjunctiva, fever of low degree (104–107 °F), dry or semidry dung, anaemia.

PM Findings: Punched-out ulcers with blood tinged base are found in abomasums, enlarged lymph nodes, pale mucosa are also seen.

Treatment: *Berenil* (MSD/intervet product). I have found it to be the best drug for treatment of theileriasis although it is also effective against Babesia and Trypanosoma and for treating pyrexia of unknown origin. Vials of 30 and 90 ml are available.

Contents: Diminazine aceturate 70 mg and phenazone 375 mg.

Dose: 5 to 10 ml per 100 kg BW. For resistant types give 10 ml/100 kg BW as deep IM injection.

Other similar drugs used are: Trityl (Lyka); Batrynil (Zydus); Prozomin (Virbac); Zokil (Mankind)

Prevention: Theileria vaccine; Rakshavec

Rakshavac-T vaccine is recommended for prophylactic vaccination against Theileriosis caused by theileria annulata in crossbred and exotic cattle. Rakshavac-T contains live schizonts grown in lymphoblast cell culture, attenuated by prolonged *in vitro* passage. Attenuated schizonts do not produce the clinical disease. Immunised cattle can withstand the attack of infected ticks for a period of three years. In areas where the vaccinated animals are constantly exposed to tick bites, the immunity is constantly boosted and hence the immunity is conferred for life time. Where the animals are maintained in tick free condition, revaccination every 3 years is recommended.

Administration

Remove the vial from liquid nitrogen container and thaw the vaccine concentrate in lukewarm (37°C) water. Transfer the thawed vaccine concentrate using a sterile needle and syringe to the corresponding vaccine diluent vial and mix gently. The reconstituted vaccine should be injected subcutaneously through an area of clean dry skin with precautions taken against contamination. The recommended site for inoculation is midneck region.

Concentrate Diluent Vaccine Volume

5 Dose 13.0 ml, 15.0 ml

Dosage

Cattle and Calves 3.0 ml.

Vaccination Regimen

Cattle and calves of 2 months age and above only should be vaccinated. Vaccination of animals in advanced stage of pregnancy should be avoided.

Immunity generally develops 6 weeks after vaccination. No other vaccine should be administered for a period of 8 weeks after Theileriasis vaccine.

Packing

Vaccine concentrate: Vials of 5 doses.

Diluent: Vials of 13 ml

Homoeopathic treatment: In Theileriasis or PUO of chronic relapsing type, give Natrum mur 1000, 1/2 teaspoonful once a day in clean mouth with a little water. Repeat if necessary.

■ TRYPANOSOMIASIS (SURRA)

Trypanosomiasis is a disease affecting all domestic animals. Causal blood protozoa is *Trypanosoma evansi*. Even tigers have died due to trypanosomiasis in Nandan Kanan zoo of Odisha, India. In camels, the disease is called "Tibarsa" because it lasts for 3 years. The disease was detected in India in 1880 and the parasite was named *T. evansi*.

Transmission

The disease is more common in hot and humid season and areas, usually from August to September because flies (Tabanus, Haematopota, and Stomoxys) multiply in such conditions. Transmission is mechanical by mouth parts of the biting flies. As many as 70% of animals in an area may get infected.

Pathogenesis

T. evansi multiply in blood and are found outside RBCs or WBCs. They may localise in CNS producing anaemia and nervous symptoms, such as paraplegia, paralysis convulsions and circling. Abortions occur in pregnant animals. In camels and horses, it is highly fatal. Oedema of dependant parts of body is common.

Treatment

1. *Nilbery Injection* (Neovet/Intas) contains Diminazine Diaceturate 70 mg + Phenazone 375 mg. This is also effective against Babesia. Dose is 3.5 to 7.5 mg/kg BW or 1 ml/10–20 kg BW; deep IM.
2. *Batrynil (Zydus product)* Same as Nilbery in all respects. Injections of multiple sites is better.
3. *Prozomin* (Virbac): Same as above 2 drugs.
4. *Antrycide injection (Virbac)*: Qunapyramine sulphate and chloride (15 ml diluents + 2.5 g drug). It is preventive and curative. Dose is 2 ml per 45 kg but by SC route at multiple sites (shoulder, dewlap, and cauded fold).

Diagnosis

1. Blood smears stained by Giemsa preferably during high fever show elongated flagellated parasites between the blood cells.
2. Centrifuge blood with anticoagulant in capillary tubes of michrohematocrit centrifuge and the buffy layer is examined at low or high power (Woo's method) or as wet preparation under dark ground microscope (Murray's method).
3. Other methods of diagnosis are indirect immunofluorescent (IFAT) examination of smears.
4. Capillary agglutination test and ELISA.

Prophylaxis: Antrycide injection (Virbac) is also preventive at a dose rate of 7.4 mg/kg BW SC. The biting flies may be controlled by insecticide sprays or fly repellents.

Trityl Injection (Lyka: contains Diminazine aceturate 70 mg + Phenazone 375 mg. Active against Babesia, trypanosome, theileria and in PUO. Dose for cattle, buffaloes, sheep, goat and dogs is 1 ml per 10 kg BW by deep IM injection.

Zokill-RTU (Mankind): Composition as for Trityl, etc. Packing 30 ml, 90 ml dose as above. For PUO, 5 ml/100 kg BW by IM or SC.

Control of ticks: Control of ticks is essential to control babesiosis and other haemo-protozoa.

A list of drugs is given below:

Virtraz (Amitraz) of Virbac: It controls ticks, mites, lice and kids in all domestic animals including dogs. (6, 15, and 50 ml packs). 2 ml per litre of water is applied over the affected parts as one application per week. It is also used for humpsore and earsore, an ulcerating, bleeding parasitic condition.

Clinar: It contains cypermethrin 10% w/v. Add 1–2 ml Clinar liquid in 1 litre of water and apply thoroughly on the body. If there is a heavy problem, repeat application after 1 hour. For heavy treatment spray 20 ml Clinar mixed in 5 litre water. This should also be spreayed in cracks, crevices, barks of trees and all possible hiding places. Presentation 5, 15, 50 ml, ad 1 litre packing. (Use rubber gloves while using).

▦ TIKKIL (INDIAN IMMUNOLOGICALS LTD)

Contains 1% Cypermethrin (available as 100 ml pet bottle)—For pets 25–50 ml is sprayed as for Clinar.

▦ ECTENDOPARASITICIDAL DRUGS

These drugs kill not only ectoparasites but also endoparasites.

Zycloz bolus and injections

Oral solution contains 150 mg Closantel/ml.

Bolus: Contains 1–6 g Closantel.
Injection—100 mg per ml.

Use: In all domestic animals including pets.

Endoparasites: Haemonchus, Bunostornum, Ancylostoma, Oesophagostomum, Fasciola sp, and Schistosoma.

Ectoparasites: All types of ticks, Gastrophilus and Melophagus ovis, Oestrus ovis larvae, round and tapeworms.

Dose: Injection of 1 ml/20 kg BW or 1 ml oral/15 kg BW; bolus/100 kg BW.

▦ CANINE EHRLICHIOSIS

Ehrlichia canis and *Ehrlichia platys* cause tropical canine pancytopenia due to its affinity/target of bone marrow cells including thrombocytes. It is a silent killer because it causes damage in early subclinical stage. When it is diagnosed, it is too late for treatment.

Canine granulocytic ehrlichiosis is caused by Anaplasma phagocytophilam.

Morphology

Rickettsia are rod-shaped, coccoid or dipplococcus-shaped or often pleomorphic bacteria. It is seen in Indian dogs also, particularly in German Shephard dogs and greyhounds.

Infection

Ticks carry the disease and transmit it by bites. Infection can also pass on by blood transfusion. Incubation period of 8–20 days is followed by:
- Acute phase: of 1 to 4 weeks.
- Subclinical phase: 6–9 weeks postinfection.
- Chronic phase: after 6–9 weeks.

Symptoms

Acute phase: During this phase organisms multiply within the blood cells and spread to all areas of the body, producing fever, lethargy, loss of appetite and weight. Most important signs which lead to diagnosis are bleeding from nose and under the skin producing red patches like bruises, pain and stiffness (due to arthritis and bleeding in muscles; coughing and discharge from eyes and nose), vomiting, diarrhoea, and conjunctivitis. The effect on nervous system includes incoordination, depression, paralysis, etc.

Subclinical phase: 6–9 weeks after infection. Dogs with good immunity may recover from acute phase. Otherwise weakness, unthriftiness, anaemia is seen. On blood examination there is fall in haemoglobin, total platelet count, low WBCs and RBCs (neutropenia, eosinopenia). Blood smears show blue to purple colonies or morulae in group to 5 to 7 or several hundred coccoid organisms (0.2 to 0.5 μ diameter) in the cytoplasm of leucocytes in Giemsa stained smears). Rickettsial colonies and perivascular cuffing are seen in endothelial cells of brain. Do not forget the presence of ticks in skin (early phase). Nephrosis leads to vomiting due to uraemia and presence of protein in urine, convulsions due to uraemia and lastly, kidney failure.

Chronic Phase: Clinical signs are variable including bleeding abnormalities, specially from nose.

Blood examination shows high globulin level, low plasma albumin, thrombo-cytopenia and leucopenia.

Treatment

1. Tetracyclin or doxycyclin administered for at least 3 weeks is the method of choice. Tetracyclin, 20 mg kg/IM for 5 days initially.
   Oxytetracyclin (10 mg/kg/IV daily) during acute phase is effective but infection is not eliminated (Oxytetracyclin, L.A. of Zydus is good).
   Trimethoprim and sulfadimidine and sulfamethylphenazole (20 and 50 mg with 50 mg/kg BW respectively can be tried) Oriprim injection of Zydus is also good. Relapse can occur.
2. *Haematonics:* Iron tonics. I use Feriate (iron + sucros) of Lucid Pharmaceuticals
   Control: Injection (20 mg/ml). It is diluted with normal saline to contain 2 mg in 1 ml IV infusion is slowly done in 15 minutes. Sharkofernol oral (Alembic) can also be given. Treatment against ticks is the wisest step.

▩ TICK BORNE FEVER OR EHRLICHIOSIS (RUMINANTS)

Cause: Anaplasma phagocytophila

Hosts: Cattle, sheep and goats

Signs: Fever (often diagnosed as pyrexia of unknown origin or PUO), depression, lethargy, high respiratory rate or abortions.

Clinical Pathology

Thrombocytopenia, later prolonged neutropenia and lymphocytopenia.

Diagnosis

Demonstration of *Anaplasma phagocytophila (Ehrlichia phagocytophila)* obligate intracellular parasite, *Anaplasma (Ehrlichia) bovis* in cattle.

Anaplasma can be detected as intracytoplasmic inclusion bodies in neutrophil cytoplasm in acute phase by Giemsa staining of blood smears.

Treatment

As given above. Oxytetracycline injections are best (10 mg/kg/IV, daily) in acute phase. In goats good results are obtained by oxytetracycline (10 mg/kg/IV) as a single dose or by sulpha drugs mentioned above (trimethoprim and sulfadimidine). Give nutritional supplements, haematonics and liver tonics to prevent jaundice.

Note: It seems that the cases of Ehrlichiosis in dogs, calves, goats and pigs, particularly in dogs and calves remain undiagnosed by field veterinarians and they may pass it on as Pyrexia or unknown origin or PUO or the doctors may grope in the dark for treatment. It is therefore pointed out that they should suspect this disease on the following basis:

1. If there are or there were ticks in the animal
2. Fever onset, bleeding from nose, and skin, etc.
3. If 'a' and 'b' are positive, go for detecting:
   - Thrombocytopenia (low platelet count) + enlarged lymph nodes and spleen
   - Presence of purple colonies or morulae or coccoid bodies in the cytoplasm of blood cells.
   - Leukopenia, anaemia (pale conjunctiva and oral/nasal mucosa)
   - High globulin level in chronic cases

If suspected for Ehrlichiosis, immediately start:

1. Tetracyclin or doxycyclin injections (long spell of 2 to 3 weeks, 10 mg/kg/IV daily for 5–6 weeks). Doxycyclin only orally in dogs.
2. Other measures given under treatment.
3. *Tranexamic acid (TXA) sold as 'Texableed'*, a product of Vet Mankind, New Delhi at the rate of 8 mg/kg BW IM twice daily to control bleeding. It is antifibrinolytic drug and safe.
4. Prednisolon 1 mg/kg BW IM for 10 days may be injected to improve platelet count. (Sarita Devi et al, Intas Polvet, 2015, 16. 350-352).
5. Adrenalin may be used as intranasal tempons (gauze) as topical haemostatic.
6. Supportive therapy: Injections of liver extract (Belamyl and anabolic steroid *nandrolone or Cypon syrup orally).*
7. *Nandrolone* (Intas Pharma) 1 mg/kg BW, IM every 1–2 weeks.
8. *Morbofloxacin eyedrops* and vitamin B complex syrup.
9. *'Pet Spark'* of Venkey's Pet, 5–10 ml twice a day is very good. It contains vitamins (for dogs), 200 ml pack.
10. *Ventriliv Pet of* Venkey's Pet: Contains Selymerin and choline chloride ond 7 hepatoprotectants: Give 5–10 ml twice a day (in dogs).
11. *Yakrifit or Liv 52;* 20–25 ml twice a day for 7 days.

Homoeopathic support for Ehrlichiosis

1. Phosphorus 200 liquid 10 ml or 30 ml: Give 10 drops three times a day.
2. Arsenicum album 1000: Give 10–15 drops by mouth once a day.
3. Natrum mur 1000: 4–6 drops in 3 days (in dogs and calves).

All dogs start taking food after 10 to 12 hours. Recovery expected after 1 month.
Monitoring recovery: By clinical signs, appetite, and blood parameter.
Blood parameters (Sarita Devi et al, 2015).

	Before treatment values	Afer treatment values (2 weeks)
Haemoglobin	4.7–5.3 G/DL	10.3–11.2
PCV	15–17%	31–36
Platelets (cmm)	92000–1, 32,000	2,02,000–3, 20,000
ALT (alanin amino transferase)	86.6–98.1	45.4–51.3
AST	72–174.2	39.3–45.2 (liver repair)

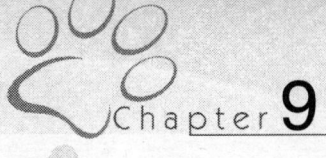

Chapter 9

Parasitic Diseases of Cattle, Sheep, Goat and Dog

There are several dozens of roundworms, tapeworms, trematodes and cestodes affecting ruminants besides dozens of ectoparasites. I am not dealing with all parasites but dealing with endoparasites (within the body) as a single problem because all of them can be prevented and treated by any of the several antiparasitic drugs. Blood protozoa have been dealt with separately.

I am, however, highlighting the most important and economically important parasitic diseases which I have seen in the cattle, sheep and goats in my 12 years' practice with ruminants.

■ HAEMONCHOSIS

Cattle, sheep, and goats: Haemonchus (*H. babalis, H. contortus, H. placei*) and *Bunostomum* sp—all are blood sucking worms found in abomasums. *H. contortus* is found in abomasums of goats and sheep. Bunostomum are red worms attached to small intestine of cattle, sheep and goats. All these produce up to 10,000 eggs each and have direct life cycle, therefore, they pose a serious herd problem. All suck blood hence there can be serious anaemia resulting in pallor of mucosa (conjunctiva), unthriftiness, alkaline indigestion. Presence of 355 worms which suck blood may bring haemoglobin to as low as 8 g/dl. 'Bottle jaw' may be seen due to hypo-proteinemia. One worm sucks 0.05 ml blood per day.

Treatment

By broad-spectrum anthelmintics such as *Lymec CN injection* (Lyka). This not only kills haemonchus sp. But also lung worms, filaroid worms, liver flukes and external parasites, mites, lice, ticks and skin larvae due to myiasis. Packing is of 10 ml. Contents: Ivermectin, clorsulon in some alcohol.

Dose: Cattle/buffalo: 1 ml/50 kg BW.

Sheep and goats: 0.5 ml/25 kg BW as SC injection.

Hitek-F: Contains ivermectin + clorsulon; injection (10 ml vial) by Virbac. Dose and route are as described above.

Hitek alone injection (10, 30 ml by Virbac): Contains ivermectin and protects also for 14 days. Repeat deworming if required monthly.

Other companies use injections containing closantel refoxanide or nitroxynil with ivermectin which kills liver flukes also. Orally ivermectin or albendazol may be used.

Diagnosis

Directly seeing thin wireworms, wriggling like snakes when contents of abomasums are mixed with clear water. In sheep and goats see the worms carefully because of the small size. Fecal examination shows eggs.

Ostertagia, Trichostrongylus, and Strongyloides

These worms also infect digestive system but do not suck blood. They produce diarrhoea, dullness, anorexia, and anaemia. These worms also are treated by above medicines. Anaemia (degree) is examined by matching conjunctiva with graded colour chart in USA, Australia and other countries.

■ OESOPHAGOSTOMIASIS (NODULAR OR PIMPLY GUT DISEASE)

This is the most common disease I have seen in sheep and goats which results in serious damage to intestine by formation of pea-sized nodules. Species of oesophagostomum are:

O. columbianum, O. venulosum, etc. in sheep and goats; *O. venulosum* and *O. radiatum* in cattle.

Symptoms

- Anorexia
- Persistant mucoid diarrhoea
- Loss of weight
- Hypoproteinemia
- Death—even by 200 worms.

Lesions: Yellowish nodules with pus and larva are found in colon with catarrhal colitis. Nodules may progress to peritonitis or even bleeding from intestine.

Diagnosis

At postmortem by 'pimply gut' low serum protein and anaemia.

Treatment

As for haemonchus and ostertagia.

■ ASCARIS WORMS

Common roundworms of animals.

Cause

Parascaris vitulorum. Hosts are calves of cattle and buffaloes. Worms are 20–50 cm long and round. In adult, the larvae remain dormant and are passed out about the calving period and passed out in milk. The larvae while passing through liver and lungs produce hepatitis and pneumonia.

Symptoms

Diarrhoea without fever. Sometimes obstructive jaundice. In small calves spasms in legs are observed due to neurotoxin.

Diagnosis

Characteristic eggs are seen in faeces.

Treatment

By common dewormins and oral medicines such as albendazol (Minthol bolus of Alembic)

Fenbendazole 0.5 mg/kg BW can be given.

Ivermectin: 0.2 mg/kg BW orally (Currminth of Zydus).

Mebendazole: 5–10 mg/kg BW orally or injections described for haemonchosis (Lymec and Hitek).

Piperazine (Bripazine of Brihans Lab): This is cheap and effective drug which is manufactured by almost all reputed drug companies.

Dose: 100–400 mg/kg BW in cattle and horses.

Levamisole: 10 mg/kg BW.

Zyclozz (Zydus) contains Closantel: Kills most of ecto and endoparasites, available in injection, bolus, and liquid form.

Life cycle: Ascaris have direct life cycle.

Eggs → Faeces → Food/Water → Host → Larvae (liver) → Lungs → Intestines
(total about 2 months' time)

Prevention

1. Proper disposal of cow dung or faeces.
2. Regular deworming.
3. Deworming of pregnant cows before parturition.

Endact Plus: Ivermactine + Clorsulon (product of Vetoquinol India)—Dose same as given for Neomac sx.

Panacur (MSD/Intervet product): Contains Fenbendazole 250 mg/8 g; 6 g, 60 g, and 120 g sache are available.

Dose: 5 mg Fenbendazole/kg BW. Mix 6 g in 100 ml, 60 g in 1 litre, and 120 g in 2 litres of water. It is effective against all roundworms including oesophagostomum, neoascaris, haemonchus, lungworms, ancylostoma in dogs, hyostrongylus, trichuris, tapeworms, etc. Give 5 mg fenbendazole per kg BW.

Fensafe: Fenbendazloe + ivermectin 3 g + 100 mg respectively (Hester) in one bolus. Dose: 3 bolus per 400 kg BW (orally)

Flukines-L (Neospark): Contains Trichobendazole + Levamisole 0.5 and 1 litre. Dose: 2 ml/10 kg BW. It is good also against larva.

▇ TAPEWORMS

Tapeworms are long, white, tapelike, segmented worms. They are found only in the intestine in India and Mediterranean countries. Important ones are:

Moniezia expansa and *M. benedini*: Hosts are cattle, buffaloes, sheep and goats

Anoplocephala sp are found in horses.

Pathogenesis

Tapeworms are poorly pathogenic. Their eggs are found in segments. Infection occurs after eating pasture mites. The affected adult animals are mostly sympomless but young calves may show diarrhoea and poor health.

Treatment

1. *Albendazol* as described above. 5–7 mg per kg BW.
2. *Praziquantel + Pyrental pamoate + Fenbendazole,* 50 + 144 + 500 mg respectively (Prazital Forte of Indian Immunologicals Ltd) which eliminates hookworms, roundworms, and tapeworms.
   Dose: 1 tablet per 10 kg, orally.
3. *Fensafe 3000* (Hester product): dose given above as bolus.
4. *Plozin (Pfizer product)* 1 tablet x box of 12 strips.
   Contains Fenbendazole, praziquintel and pyrental pamoate (500 + 50 + 144 mg respectively).
   Dose: Give orally 1 tablet per 10 kg BW. Give Plozin Plus.
5. *Prazisum Plus* (Vetoquinol): It kills all intestinal worms and also Hydatid worms
   Dose: 1 tablet/ 10 kg BW.

Tonics: It is advisable to give any of the liver and B complex tablets or syrup to make the animal withstand the stress of deworming (e.g. Kepoliv of Kepler, 300 ml or 1 litre bottle).

Dose: Cows and buffaloes—30 ml daily; calves, sheep and goats—15 ml daily.

NASAL MYIASIS IN SHEEP

The larvae of *Oestrus ovis* are deposited in the nose of sheep and sometimes in goats of 3–5 years age. Mucopurul ent nasal discharge and too much sneezing are the main symptoms. The larvae are 1.5 to 2 cm long, curved, and have 2 hooks by which they attach to the nasal mucosa.

Treatment

1. *Ivermectin* (Neomec) 200 mg/kg BW/SC injection, weekly for 4 weeks.
2. *Enrofloxacin and bromhexidine hydrochloride* 10 mg/kg BW for 5 days to remove infection of bacteria in sinuses.
3. *Prednisolon 5* mg/kg BW for 3 days.
   Recovery starts by 5th day.

LUMBAR PARALYSIS (CEREBROSPINAL NEMATODIASIS)

Cerebrospinal nematodiasis means a condition in which nematode larvae migrate abnormally into the brain and spinal cord. Main larvae which do so are larvae of (Setaria sp) filarid worms found in the peritoneal cavity of ruminants. This abnormal migration of larvae in CNS results in lumbar paralysis more often seen in sheep and goats. Such sheep and goats show lumbar weakness, incoordination of hindlimbs, wobbling and sometimes paralysis. Similar symptoms may also be seen due to warble fly larvae or rabies in sheep.

Although cure is not guaranteed, antihelminthic drugs such as ivermectin may kill the larvae and prevent further damage. Ivermectin injected twice at the dose rate of 0.2 mg/kg BW may help in lumbar paralysis along with injection of *'Nuroxin M'* (Zydus product) and *Vetakey injection of Zydus* (containing multivitamin + choline + phosphorus, etc). These drugs will help in remyelination. Similar condition called *'Kumri'* also occurs in horses in India.

■ HOOKWORMS

Hookworms are small nematodes which attach to stomach or intestinal wall and suck blood, causing anaemia in all species. About 2000 hookworms may kill a young cattle. The important hookworms are listed below.

Name of worm	Host	Importance for India
Ancylastoma caninum	Dogs, wolf	Yes
A. Ceylanicum	Dogs, cats	Not important
A. Tubaeforme	Cats	important
Bunostomum sp	Cattle	important

Symptoms

Severe anaemia, creeping eruptions. This condition means blood stained linear lesions in skin, causing itching.

Treatment

Approach for treatment is the same as described for haemonchus worms. Calves of 4–12 months age are more commonly affected.

■ HEARTWORMS IN DOGS

Heartworms called *Dirofilaria immitis* are important. I have recorded this condition in Jharkhand and Gujarat but may be seen in any other state also.

These nematodes are fairly big, up to several centimeters long and are found in the right ventricle and produce larvae and not eggs called microfilaria. Mosquitoes ingest microfilaria and transmit them to new dogs or cats.

Symptoms

Breathing problem, weakness, cardiac dilation, ascites (due to passive venous congestion). Dead worms may cause pulmonary embolism. Death is due to cardiac failure.

Diagnosis

A test kit using a conjugate for detection of antigen in serum of suspected dog. The test is a simple immunodiffusion test on the test plate which gives test result by coloured band in the test plate (Imported from Germany called IDEXX Kit). Heart damage kit called SD Troponin are regulatory proteins produced in the heart muscles (Available from M46-47, Phase III B, Verma industrial area, Goa -403722, India).

Treatment

For prevention, ivermectin (such as Ivectin of Indian Immunologicals) 6 mg/kg/month can be given orally. Lymec or Hitek injections of ivermectins of (Lyka and Virbac) can also be used.

Piperazine such as Lyzine of Lyca and Peperazine 45% of TTK can kill the worms but may result in embolism in the lungs.

Homoeopathy: heart drops R# of Reckeweg Co—10 drops 3 times a day to tonne up the heart.

■ FILARIAL DERMATITIS (CUTANEOUS FILARIASIS)

This condition of skin is caused by Parafilaria multipapillosa or *P. bovicola*. The larvae are deposited by biting flies in the skin of more than 4 months old cattle, mostly in warm season. 7 to 9 months after infection (deposit) small nodules develop in the skin which break open and release adult worms along with blood. The nodules are mostly seen on shoulders, neck, around eyes, and in dulep.

Treatment: Levamisole 12 mg/kg daily for 4 days (fasnil of Merial Co or Dosch)

■ SCHISTOSOMIASIS (NASAL GRANULOMA)

It is caused by parasite *Schistosoma nasalis* and *S. bovis*. In India, it is found in many parts of India particularly in eastern states, wet areas like Chhattisgarh, Orissa, Bihar, etc. where snails, the intermediate hosts, are found.

Pathology and symptoms

The male and the female live together in the veins of nasal mucosa of cattle, sheep, goats, horses. In man, the larvae penetrate skin, causing dermatitis.

Symptoms include mucopurulent nasal discharge, formation of pustules in nose, at times bleeding from nose and most important is the 'snoring sound', particularly audible at night (snoring disease). Diagnosis is easy by finding boomerang shaped eggs having spine at one end in nasal exudates.

Treatment

1. *Anthiomaline (Lithium antimony tartrate)* 6% solution: 20 ml is injected by deep IM route in cattle and 15–20 ml in horses.
2. *Tartar emetic: 1–2% solution* is injected at the rate of 2 mg/kg BW for 6 days by IM route.
3. *Sodium antimony tartrate:* 2 mg/kg BW in 10% dextrose is injected IV, twice a day for two days. Ant. Potassium tartrate is available from HiMedia Laboratories.
4. *Antimosan:* 1.7 mg/kg BW for 6 days.
5. Distozole: Oxyclozanide + Levamisole (Neospark) liquid 100 and 500 ml pack. *Dose:* 10 ml per 20 kg BW, orally.
6. *Praziquantel:* Inject 20 mg/kg BW as a single SC injection.

■ AMPHISTOMES

Amphistomes are flukes which have suckers at both the ends of the body. They also require snails to complete the life cycle. Mature flukes, about 6–10 mm in size, pink in colour are found attached to ruminal walls but are not much harmful. The immature metacercaviae remain in duodenum for 1/2 to 4 months, producing severe enteritis and diarrhoea. Diarrhoeic faeces is foul smelling. Diarrhoea kills the host cow, buffaloes, sheep or goats in 2 to 3 weeks. There may be oedema producing 'bottle jaw' condition in late stage. There is anorexia and less of appetite.

Treatment

Give symptomatic treatment for diarrhoea. Homeopathic drug 'podophylum' 1/2 to 1 teaspoonful 2–3 times a day can give good results. Podophylum works well in diarrhoea with foul smell.

Distozole-L (Neospark) contains oxyclozanide and levamisole and is available in 100 ml, 0.5 litre, 1 litre packs. Dose: 30 ml/100 kg BW; Flukes, Amphistomes and *Moniezia expansa* (tapeworm in horses) are killed by oral dosing.

Verma Rid Forte: Rafoxanide and Levamisole combination (Neospark). Packing of 100 ml, 0.5 litre, 1 litre. Dose: 1 ml per 4 kg BW, orally.

Flukinex (Neospark) Trichobendazole 5% (Neospark) pack of 0.5 litre and 1 litre. Dose: 10 ml per 25 kg BW, orally.

Bena Mid (Neospark): Niclosamide and albendazole, 0.5 litre, 1 litre packing. Dose: 10 ml per 15 kg BW, orally.

Distodin (Zydus): Kills Amphistomes and liver fluke (tablets and bolus).

Dose: 1 bolus /100 kg BW/day, orally.
          1 tablet/ 13 kg BW/day, orally.

▣ LIVER FLUKE

Fasciola hepatica and *Fasciola gigantic* are the important liver flukes.

Hosts

Cattle, sheep, goats of hilly areas (*F. hepatica*). *F. gigantic* is more common in wet lands, around ponds, water bodies, etc. where snails, the intermediate hosts also survive. Eggs produce larva miracidium which invade snails in which redia and thousands of cercaria develop. Metacercaria, the infective stage wait on grass and plants to be eaten by ruminants. Most favourable time is summer.

Pathology

The disease may occur in acute, subacute or chronic form. Acute form is more common in sheep and goats, not cattle and buffaloes. Weight loss, off-feed and paller of mucosa and occasionally, blood stained discharge from nose and anus may be seen. In chronic form, anaemia, diarrhoea, and oedema of throat called 'bottle jaw' is common. In small animals, 'pot belly' condition is common.

Diagnosis

Eggs of fasciola are heavy and settle down to bottom of faecal emulsion hence take sample from bottom of the tube for microscopic examination. The eggs are oval and have a lid (operculum) at one end.

Treatment

1. *Ivermectin* + Clorsulon (e.g. 'neomac' SX of Intas Pharma). Neomac SX contains ivermectin 10 mg and clorsulon 100 mg per ml (10 ml vial). Dose: 1 ml/50 kg BW.
2. *Closal* (Alembic): Bolus and liquid. Bolus 1 gm closental sodium, liquid 150 mg/ml. effective against Fasciola sp, Haemonchas sp, Bunostomum and nasal bot of sheep (*Oestrus ovis*).

Dose: 1 ml/10 kg BW/orally; bolus 4 g/300 kg BW, orally

3. *Albendazol* (Minthol bolus of Alembic) bolusi 200, 600, 3000 mg effective against all GI, worms, lungworms, tapeworms, and 85% liverflukes.
   Dose: Cattle and buffaloes: 7.5 mg/kg BW 3000 mg for 3 days.
   Sheep and goats: 300 mg/ 40 kg BW.

4. *Fasnil (suspension, Merial/Dosch product):* Contents: Levamisol and oxyclozanide. Kills mature and immature flukes, larval and adult GI roundworms, lung worms and nasal bots (sheep and goats)

5. *Fasmin bolus and suspension (Lyka):* Dose: 1 bolus/66 kg but sheep and goat to be given 1/2 bolus. Liquid (90 ml and 1 litre): 5 ml/10 kg BW, orally; sheep/goat— 1 ml/2 kg BW.

The major groups of anthelmintics are as under (Sheela Choudhary and others loc cit 2005)

Parasites	Chemical groups	Drugs
Nematodes	Piperazines	Piperazines salts, diethylcarbamazine
	Imidazothiazoles/ Tetrahydropyrimidines	Tetramisole, levamisole/morantel, pyrantel
		Thiabendazole, mebendazole, parbendazole,
	Benzimidazoles/ Pro-benzimidazoles	Fenbendazole, oxfendazole, albendazole, Oxibendazole, cambendazole, flubendazole, Febantel, thiophante, netobimin
	Ivermectins	Ivermectin
	Organophosphates	Dichlorvos, haloxon, trichlorfon (metriphonate),
	Salicylanilides/substituted Phenols	closantel
Trematodes	Salicylanilides/substituted Phenols	Nitroxynil, rafoxanide, oxyclozanide, brotianide, diamphenethide, niclofolan, dlosnatel
	Others	Clorsulon
	Benzimidazoles	Triclabendazole, albendazole
Cestodes	Salicylanilides/ substituted phenols	Niclosamide
	Others	Praziquantel, bunamidine, arecoline

(Brander GC and Pugh DM, 1977 and Fraser CM, 1986)

The antiparasitic spectrum of Ivermectin in animals

Species	Parasites
Cattle	Adults and fourth stage larva of Haemonchus, Ostertagia, Trichostrongylus, Cooperia, Nematodirus, Dictyocaulus, Hypoderma, lice, mites, and ticks
Horses	Large strongyles (adult) (*Strongylus vulgaris, S. equines, S. edentates*, Triodontophorus spp.) small strongyles, pinworms (adults and 4th stage larva, Dictyocaulus, Habronema, Onchocerca and Gasterophilus
Sheep and goats	Gastrointestinal nematodes, lung worms, Oestrus, Hypoderma
Dogs	Toxocara, Ancylostoma, Dirofilaria (highly effective against microfilaria), lice, mites, ticks, and fleas
Pigs	Ascaris suum, Hyostrongylus, Oesophagostomum, Metastrongylus, lice and mites
Birds	*Ascaridia galli, Heterakis gallinarum*, and Capillaria spp.

Ivermectin is a wonder drug for livestock production and health of not only animals but it is also administered to 18 million people every year (Burkhari, 2000) Vet. Hhm. Toxicol. 42: 155-199).

It must, however, be remembered that haemonchus contortus, Ostertagia, Cooperia and Parascaris equorum worms may become resistant to ivermectin, hence do not use them without discrimination.

Haematology

Eosinophil count is a good indicator of parasites, especially in dogs. In healthy dogs, eosinophil count is $1.60 \pm 0.24\%$ and in parasitic infections above 4% are good indicators of ecto or endoparasites.

Deworming of Schedule for Animals and Poultry (Sheela Chaudhary, A Chahar and A. Singh 2005 (Intas Vet, 6: 177-180)

Dog	
Pup	1st: 2 weeks, repeat after 2 weeks; 2nd: 2 months
Adult dog	Once every 3 to 4 months
Pregnant bitch	2 weeks pre-whelping
Post-whelping	2 weeks post-whelping

Newly purchased pups should be dosed twice at an interval of 14 days.

Horse	
Stage (age)	*Deworming schedule*
Foal	4, 8, 16, 20, 24, 32, and 40 weeks after birth
Yearling	In spring before pulling out to pasture
Adult horse	Once every 3 to 4 months
Pregnant mare	4 weeks pre-foaling
Post-foaling	4 weeks post-foaling

If worm disease occurs (faecal examination) 3 to 4 deworming treatments of all animals on the farm at intervals of 6 weeks is recommended.

Cattle	
Stage	*Deworming schedule*
Calf	1 month age and thereafter every month
Heifer	Once every 2 months
Adult cattle	Once every 3 to 4 months
Pregnant cow	5th month of pregnancy and 2 weeks pre-calving
Post-calving	2 weeks post-calving, to be repeated twice at one month interval

Sheep/goats	
Lamb	4, 8, and 12 weeks
Adult	Once every 2 to 3 months
Pregnant ewe/doe	4th month of pregnancy and 2 weeks pre-lambing/kidding
Postpartum	4 weeks pre-lambing/kidding

Lambs/kids given anthelmintic treatment at weaning and adults dosed 2 weeks before breeding is of value. Treatments during spring and autumn are required, where precise timings depend on lambing and service dates.

Pig	
Stage (age)	*Deworming Schedule*
Young	5–6 weeks, repeat after 4 weeks
Adult pig	Once every 3 to 4 months
Pregnant sow	1 week pre-farrowing
Post-farrowing	5–6 weeks post-farrowing

Thumb rules for deworming

1. Treat all animals in a group with anthelmintic at the same time.
2. To avoid anthelmintic resistance, never underdose an animal.
3. Frequency of drenching to be reduced as far as practicable.
4. Rotate the anthelmintic class, both between the drenches and annually.
5. After each dosing, the stock should be moved to a clean pasture which has been rested at least 4 weeks.
6. Alternative grazing—where both cattle and sheep are present alternating grazing of fields on an annual basis with each host is useful. If goats are also present, it will be advisable to allow goats first, followed by cattle and sheep in that order.
7. Rotational grazing—the susceptible younger animals should be grazed ahead followed by the immune adults.
8. Avoid grazing of animals in the same area for several successive months.
9. Reduce snail population in the environment and prevent livestock from drinking standing water supplies such as ponds.
10. Larval tapeworms are more resistant and hence it is advisable to repeat dosing at 2–3 weeks interval.
11. Animals should be adequately fed with a well-balanced diet. Diet rich in protein, vitamin A and B complex induces resistance to infection.
12. Eliminate raw fish/meat from the diet and follow thorough washing of green vegetables before including them in the diet (dogs and cats).
13. Prompt removal and suitable disposal of faeces, especially of the older animals.
14. Keep sheds, barns, stalls, etc. as clean as possible and certainly dry.

It is realised that under Indian conditions, many of the recommendations made above may not be possible, at least for the marginal farmers. In such cases, it would be preferable to give an anthelmintic course at regular intervals since the cost of the drug is comparatively small.

▓ CANINE LEPTOSPIROSIS

Cause

Leptospira interrogans (Serogroup autumnalis) is most prevalent, followed by *L. icterohaemorphagiae, L. canicola, L. Pomona,* and *L. pyrogens.* This has emerged as a serious global leptospirosis or Spirochaetal, zoonotic problem. It is often undiagnosed (Iqball et al. 2011, Indian Pet J) and remains a problem despite vaccination. In South India, it is endemic. Cases are rare due to vaccinations.

Culture

In Difco liquid culture medium or Leptospira Medium of HiMedia HiVeg (Cat. No. MV 239).

Diagnostic Test

Microscopic agglutination test (MAT) which has a bettery of six pathogenic serogroups is available from Zoonosis Research Laboratory, Tanuvas, Madhavaram, Chennai. Test sera are diluted to 1 : 50 and then serially 1 : 100—1 : 1600 in PBS. 20 µl of serum and 20 µl of antigen (live) are mixed, incubated at 37°C for 2 hours. The mixture is then examined in dark field microscope. The highest serum dilution which agglutinates 50% or more of leptospira is the titer. Titers due to vaccination are low and even.

Symptoms

Acute, subacte and chronic forms of disease are seen. In acute form, fever and anaemia lead to suspected disease. In chronic form, stillbirth, abortions, infertility, weak neonates, periodic ophthalmia may be seen.

In dogs, haemorrhages, *liver dysfunction* and *jaundice* are common. Rat (urine) is the common source of infection. Subacute form is generally due to *L. canicola* and subacute nephritis is more common, which may lead to fatal uraemia. In peracute form, bloody diarrhoea, vomiting and jaundice are more common along with fever. Peracute form is more common in puppies. In nephritic form (Stuttgart Disease), breath has uraemic smell.

Diagnosis

Simple diagnosis is possible by demonstration of spiral-shaped, motile, organisms, clearly seen in the sinusoids, and urine in early stage of the disease. For diagnosis, dark field microscopic examination of urine sediment is best to show snakelike, live organisms. Organisms may also be seen in aspirated fluid from enlarged lymph nodes.

Staining smears by silver staining method (Levadity Method) demonstrates black coloured, coiled organisms in oil emersion objective.

Prevention

Rats must be controlled to prevent entry of infection.

Vaccination

See the vaccines used for:
1. Leptospira under 'Other Virus Diseases of Dogs'. 9 in 1 vaccine (Vanguard Plus 5 L4 Vaccine of Zoetis, USA).
2. *Canigen DHPPi/L Vaccine:* This contains freeze-dried antigen: Distemper, adenovirus, parvovirus, canine parainfluenza virus, *Leptospira interrogans L canicola, Licterohaemorrhagiae* antigens.
   Use: Preventive for all above pathogens
   Inject DHPPi/L one dose vaccine by SC or IM route as per vaccination schedule at 8 and 12 weeks age.
3. *Canine Leptospirosis vaccine LEPTO (MSD):* Imported and marketed by Intervet India Pvt Ltd, Pune. Storage at 2–8°C. contains *L. canicola,* and *L. icterohaemorrhagiae* inactivated.
   Vaccinations: 8–9 weeks—Novivac DHPPi and Nobivac Lepto
   12 weeks—Novivac DHPPi and Nobivac Lepto or Nobivac RL
For other details, follow manufacturer's instructions.

Use: Shake well before use. Give SC injection in neck or chest region.

Life: Storage life is 21 months.

4. *Megavac 6:* It is live attenuated + killed antigens vaccine of Indian Immunologicals (Hyderabad)

Live attenuated part	Killed components
Canine distemper virus	Canine adenovirus type 1
Canine parvovirus	Canine adenovirus type 1
Canine adenovirus type 2	*Leptospira canicola, L icterohaemorrhagiae*

Vaccine presentation: Monopack and tray (multiple) pack

Vaccination Schedule for Leptospirosis:

1. 2 months
2. 3 months (1 month after first vaccination)
3. 4 months (1 month after second vaccination)
4. Annual vaccination

Dose: Reconstituted freeze-dried leptospira vaccine by the liquid provided with the vaccine. Inject 1 ml by SC or IM route.

Treatment

The main aim of treatment is to control the organisms before they damage vital organs, mainly liver and kidneys. The drug of choice is dihydrostreptomycin or tetracyclines, e.g. Steclin injection (Zydus) available as 30, 50, and 100 ml can be injected at the rate of 1–2 ml per 10 kg BW, IM, IV, or SC.

Steclin (Zydus) 50 mg—dose 1–2 ml 25 kg BW IM, IV, or SC.

Leptospira are also highly usceptible to ampicillin, amoxicillin, penicillin G, cephotaxime, erythromycin, and ciprofloxacin. Doxycycline and penicillin are effective in treating acute leptospirosis. To stop serious bleeding in acute form Adchrome injection can be used.

Dicrysticin S and Dicrysticin DS

DS = vial—streptomycin 5 g

Procain pen. G 30,00,000 units

Penicillin G Sod. 10,00,000 units

Dose: Large animal 2 ml/50 kg BW

Small animal 1 ml/5 kg BW

After dissolving in 7.5 ml distilled water

Homoeopathy: Give Phosph 200 in dogs, 4 drops TDS

Arsen. Alb. 1000—dogs 4 drops morning and evening

Jondilla: 1 teaspoonful TDS for dogs

Liv-T (SBL) Syrup—2 teaspoonfuls 3 times a day.

Kalmegh Liver formula (JVS)—10 drops in water 3 times.

Chapter 10

Fungal Infection in Animals

■ DERMATOPHYTOSIS (DERMATOMYCOSIS, TINEA INFECTION, RINGWORM)

Hosts and Etiology

- *Horse and cattle:* Trichophyton species
- *Dog: Microsporum canis, M. gypsium, M. mentagrophytes*
- *Man:* Trichophyton and Microsperum

Transmission

Direct or indirect contact with infected animal or even by air. Fungal spores can exist for a long-time on skin of animals without producing disease. The infection is confined to dead layers of skin or hairs.

Lesions

In dogs, skin of face is a common site although it can occur elsewhere also. Mostly skin around nostrils is affected, then of neck may be affected. Lesons are around 1–4 mm or larger in size. In dogs, there is alopecia, scale formation and crust formation.

Treatment and Control

For prevention, 2% formalin or 1% caustic soda (NaOH) may be applied on the doors and windows, walls, ropes, chains, etc. to kill the contaminating fungus.

1. *Sheen-n-Kleen Forte (Pfizer)* which contains ketoconazole and chlorhexidine gluconate, is applied as a shampoo on wet skin of pets and washed after 7 to 10 minutes.
2. *Myconil (dual protector)*: It treats keratoseborrhoeic disorders, greasy seborrhoea, *Malassezia pachydermis* (yeast) infection, staphylococcal and other bacterial infections, pyoderma (pus in skin), demodicosis and fungal infections including ringworm. (Contents ketoconazole, chlorhexidine (100 ml bottle).
3. *Pet Derm (Pfizer)*: Antibacterial, antifungal antipruritic and anti-inflammatory. Contains chlorhexidine gluconate 2% and miconazole nitrate 2%. Available as 200 ml foam and 100 ml spray.
4. *Spectrazole (Pfizer)*: Contains miconazole, ofloxacin, clobetasol. It is a cream to treat eczema, fungus, bacterial infections and wounds. Clean and apply 2–3 times a day. Available as 20, 30, and 100 g cream; 30 and 100 g lotion.
5. *Salphoben (150 ml bottle)*: Contains micronised sulphur, benzoyl peroxide and zinc oxide. Use for treating seborrhoeic problems, dandruff, dermatitis, itching, bad odour, hot (red) spots, flea bites, etc. Apply this shampoo in wet hairs, leave for 10–15 minutes and then wash well with clean water. Use till recovery.

6. *Charmil Plus* (tube and spray, 25 g, 50 g tube and 100 ml spray): Ayurvedic/herbal product which cures, manages, ringworm, dermatomycosis, eczema, and feet lesions. Apply once or twice daily till recovery.
7. *Voxeto (Intas)*: Paste, herbal. Effective to treat ringworm, eczema, dermatitis, pyoderma, pruritus, mange, maggots, and dermatomycesis.
8. *Caniderm (Rectus Remedies)*: It is a herbal product for eczema.
9. *Dermasulf ointment*: For all skin problems.
10. *Neocharm herbal paste* (Dabur).

▦ RECOMMENDATION OF ANTIMICROBIAL ADMINISTRATION IN ADULT DOGS AND PUPPIES

Drugs	Route	Adult Dogs Interval (hr) dose/mg/kg body weight	Dose puppies compared with standard adult doses	Comments	
Penicillin	*PO =oral			Increased	Minimal
Penicillin G		10,000		initial dose	adjustment
Procaine	IM, SC	20,000	12–24000 mg/kg	may lengthen	
Cloxacillin	PO, IV, IM	30	8	dose interval	
Amoxicillin	POJV,	10–20	8–12		
Ampicillin sod	PO, IVJM, SC	10–50	88		
Cephalosporins				Increased	Minimal
Cefadroxil	PO	20	12	initial dose	adjustment
Cephalexin	PO	20–30	8–12	may lengthen	
Cephradine	PO	12–20	6–8	dose interval	
Cefazolin	IV, IM, SC	10–30	6–8		
Cephapirin	IV, IM, SC	20–40	8		
Cephradine	IV, IM, SC	6–25	6–8		
Cefotaxime	IV, IM, SC	20–80	8		
Aminoglycosides				Lengthen	Avoid use in
Amikacin	IV, IM, SC	10	8	dose interval	first weeks
Dihydro-streptomycin	PO, IM, SC	10–20	612	of life	
Gentamicin	IV, JM, SC	2–4	8		
Neomycin	PO	10	6		
streptomycin	PO, IM, SC	2010	612		
Fluoroquinolones				Lengthen	Avoid use in
Ciprofloxacin	PO	5–15	12	dose interval	first weeks
Enrofloxacin	PO	2.5–15	12		of life
Norfloxacin	PO	5–20	2		
Tetracyclines				No change	
Chlortetracycline	PO	10–20	8		
Doxycycline	PO, IV	5–10	12		
Oxytetracycline	PO, IV, IM	2010	812		
Tetracycline	PO, IV, IM	2010	812		
Sulphonamides and Potentiators					
Sulfadiazine-trimethoprim	PO, IV, IM, SC	30 (combined)	12–24	Reduced dose	Avoid use in first weeks
Sulfamethoxazole-trimethoprim	PO	30 (combined)	12–14		of life

Contd...

Drugs	Route	Adult Dogs Interval (hr) dose/mg/kg body weight	Dose puppies compared with standard adult doses	Comments	
Miscellaneous Antimicrobials					
Chloramphenicol	PO, IV, IM, SC	50	8	Reduced dose	Avoid use in
Metronidazole	PO, IV	10	8		first weeks of life

Due to delayed development of renal function, a lengthening of dosage interval may produce effective tissue concentration of the drug in puppies.

Cephalosporins

The neonatal pharmacokinetics of cephalosporins are similar to those of penicillins.

Aminoglycosides

Unless special consideration is made for dosage adjustment in the neonate, the risk of adverse reactions with aminoglycoside is increased due to altered drug disposition. Aminoglycosides are excreted only through glomerular filtration which requires several weeks in newborn. Moreover, the volume of distribution is greater due to increased body water content in the neonates. Thus, half-life is lengthened and peak concentrations are high, leading to toxicity.

Chapter 11

Nerve Injuries or Degeneration

1. Neurological disorders—limping, lameness, incoordination
2. Nervine weakness—lumbar weakness, leg weakness
3. Paralysis
4. Neuromuscular disorders.

1. *Tribivet M injections* (Intas, Neovet product)
   Packing of 5 , 30 and 100 ml
   Contents: Methylcobalamin 500 mcg
            Pyridoxin HCl 50 mg
            Nicotinamide 50 mg
   Dosage: Small animals 3 to 5 ml for 3 to 6 days
   Large animals: 5 to 10 ml for 3 to 6 days.

2. *Napler: Injection* (Kepler product)
   Contents: Sod. Acid phosphate 400 mg
           Methyl cobalamin 100 mcg
   Indications: General weakness, rickets, pica, etc.
   Dose: Large animals 10 ml daily.
          Small animals 5 ml daily, IM route.

3. *Neurobion injections*: 2 ml, IM on alternate days till recovery in 15–20 days (2 ml vials)

4. *Tonoricin injection* (Vetoquinol)
   Contents: Dimethylamino-2 methylphenyl-phosphinic acid 0.2 g/ml
   Use: Treatment or prevention of hypophosphataemia and pic (eating abnormal items)
   Dose: Acute form: 1–2 ml; SC, IM, or IV route everyday for 1 to 2 weeks.

5. *Lyphos Vet* (Lyka Animal Health)
   Dogs: Lameness, incoordination, bone injury, 1–3 ml IM.

6. *Samolac* (feed supplement, Vetoquind Co): Packing of 400 g: contains vitamins, minerals, essential fatty acids and fibre. Follow directions given on container.
   Homoeopathic: Traumasol (JVS Pharma): For all types of tissue injury
   Calendula helps in regeneration; 30 ml bottle
   Give 10–20 drops diluted with some water 3 times a day till recovery (as an aid with other medicines).

■ PARALYSIS IN PETS AND CATTLE

Paralysis can be classified as:
1. Cerebral (brain lesions).

2. Spinal (damage to spinal cord).
3. Peripheral (nerve lesions).

Causes

Encephalitis, pressure of cysts, tumours, accidental, spondylopathy, slip disc, vertebral enkylosis (fusion), rheumatic, deficiency of B vitamins (B_1, B_6, and B_{12}). Injury to nerves.

Paralysis may be *spastic* (contraction of muscles or *flaccid* (nonspastic flaccid muscles).

Paraplegia means paralysis of hind quarter and hind legs. It is more common. It is of two types.

Paraplegia in extension: In this case, pyramidal tract is involved. In this case the legs are always extended and kept forward under the belly.

Paraplegia of Flexion

In this case, legs are flaccid, powerless, and drawn trailing behind the body.

Radial Paralysis

This is also called *'dropped elbow'* due to damage to radial nerve of forelimb. The animal stands without bearing weight on the leg.

Peroneal Paralysis

This is paralysis of one or both hind legs in cattle, generally after parturition due to pressure or injury in nerves passing through pelvis. This is also seen in horses. In this case, fetlock and hoofs are drawn backwards.

Management

1. Give complete rest to the animal.
2. Administer vitamin B injection (nurobion or nurokind) and calcium injections (Intalyte injection of Intas Pharma).
3. Turn the animal frequently to prevent bedsores.
4. Massage the affected part with creams containing diclofenec, etc. (such as Dynapar).
5. Infrared therapy, short durations of 2, 5 minutes.
6. Tolfenamic acid injection (Intas); 40 mg per ml; 30 and 100 ml vials. Give by IM or IV route 4 mg/kg BW. Repeat after 48 hours 2 mg/kg BW.
7. Injections of Butaphosphan + Cyanocobalamin (metabolic boosters) empowering muscles and nerves: 2.5–5 ml per 20–30 kg BW.
8. B complex injection: Mainly thiamin, pyridoxin and cyanocobalamin like tribivet (Intas): 0.5–2 ml/20–30 kg BW by IM/IV.
9. *Ascal Pet*: Oral calcium supplement (Alembic). 300 ml pet bottle
   Dose for puppy: 5 ml daily, oral
   Growning dog: 10 ml, daily, oral
   Adult dog: 20 ml daily, oral
10. *Metaphos* (Butaphosphan and mecobalamin injection —SC, IM or IV). The injection is to be given at following dose rate:
    Dogs/cats: 0.5 to 2.5 ml
    Sheep and goat: 2.5 to 8 ml
    Calf: 5 to 12 ml

For treating weakness, tetanus and paresis, anaemia, etc.

11. *Phosphovet Injections* (Dosch Pharma): To treat paraplegia.
    In acute cases: Small animals—1 to 3 ml (IM/IV)
    Chronic cases: 1 to 2 ml daily or alternate days

12. *Intacal Pet (Neovet/Intas Pharma):* Oral for pets: Pups—5 ml twice daily

13. *Beejet Injection (VetsFarma):* Boosts moto activity. Best in peroneal paralysis and supportive in dogs. Packing of 100 ml.
    Dose:
    Cattle and horse: 10 ml/day for 3–5 days
    Camel: 10–15 ml
    Goats and sheep: 3–5 ml
    Dog: 3 ml for 3 to 5 days
    Route of injection: IM, IV

■ COENUROSIS (GID OR STURDY)

This condition is caused by intermediate, cystic stage of tapeworm *Taenia multiceps*. The cystic stage is called *Coenurus cerebralis*. The tapeworm is found in dogs or wild canines. The eggs eaten from dogs' faeces by ruminants enter into the brain via blood in the form of embryos. Coenurus cysts develop in brain of sheep, goats, cattle, and horses. The cysts are about 5 cm in diameter.

Symptoms

Salivation, deviation of eye or head, moving or running about, convulsions, blindness. Going round in circles (GID) or pressing head against wall or hard objects.

Treatment

Surgical removal of the cyst, generally results in complete recovery. For prevention, taenicidal drugs must be periodically given to dogs. One of the best drugs is Prazisam Plus (Vetoquinol). Dose is 1 tablet per 10 kg BW in dogs.

Chapter 12

Urinary Diseases

URINE-NORMAL VALUES AND TESTS

	S.gravity	PH	Serum Creatinine	Serum Urea	Acid Phosphatase	Serum (SGPT)	Serum (SGOT)
Horse	1.020–1.050	8.0	0.5–1.2 mg/dl	20–40 mg/dl	1–5 IU/L	10–40 IU/L	10–40 IU/L
Cattle	1.015–1.045	7.4–8.4	0.5–1.2 mg/dl	20–40 mg/dl	1–5 IU/L	10–40 IU/L	10–40 IU/L
Sheep/ goat	As above	7.5–8.4	0.5–1.2 mg/dl	20–40 mg/dl	1–5 IU/L	10–40 IU/L	10–40 IU/L
Dog	1.020–1.045	Acid/6–7	0.5–1.2 mg/dl	20–40 mg/dl	1–5 IU/L	10–40 IU/L	10–40 IU/L
Pig	1.065–1.025	Acid/alk	0.5–1.2 mg/dl	20–40 mg/dl	1–5 IU/L	10–40 IU/L	10–40 IU/L

Cloudy urine: Due to leukocytes, erythrocytes, epithelial cells

Opaque urine: Due to bacteria, mucous, crystals.

Odour: Sweetish—ketosis

Red urine: In Bovine babesiosis

Proteins: Robert's test (Reagent)—100 ml nitric acid concentrated + 500 ml saturated magnesium sulphate.

Take 2 ml reagent, add 2 ml urine slowly, on the reagent by side of the tube. A white or cloudy ring may appear at the junction, indicating presence of albumin/protein which may be due to nephritis pyelonephritis, nephrosis, or due to congestive cardiac failure, ketosis, high fever, or starvation. Milk fever may also be present.

Ketones in urine: Rothera's test

Saturate 5 ml urine with ammonium sulphate. Add 2–3 drops of sodium nitro-prusside to the urine. Then add strong ammonium hydroxide in small quantities. If positive, a purple colour develops at the junction.

Blood in urine: Dissolve some benzidine in glacial acetic acid in a test tube. Add 2 ml urine to the above solution, then add 1 ml of fresh hydrogen peroxide. If blood is present, a bluish or bluish green colour develops.

Result: Cystitis, acute nephritis, haematuria, or haemoglobinuria.

Glucose in urine: Take 0.5 ml (8 drops) of urine in a test tube. Add 5 ml Benedict's reagent to the urine taken and mix properly. Heat near the top of the mixture then heat slowly downwards to prevent spurting of boiling mixture. Give periodical slow heat on the burner to start boiling.

- Greenish indicates (+)
- Yellows (-++)
- Red colour develops (_+++)

Result: Fear or excitement, diabetes mellitus, after general anaesthesia, shock, pulpy kidney disease, chronic liver disease. False + test with some medicines, antibiotics and ascorbic acid.

Bile salts: Hay's sulphur test: Add a pinch of yellow sulphur powder to some urine in a test tube. In positive cases, sulphur settles down to the bottom. If it floats, bile salts are absent.

Microscopic Test:

1. Take sediment of lightly centrifuged urine for microscopic examination. If RBCs are present, it indicates haematuria.
2. Presence of degenerating neutrophils indicates pus cells due to cystitis, pyelonephritis, etc.
3. *Casts:* Epithelial casts, in nephritis; RBC casts in cases of nephrosis, hyaline casts indicate protein casts in chronic nephritis, or high fever.
4. Organisms can be seen in Gram's or methylene blue (1%) stained, [dried, and fixed (by alcohol) smear] seen under oil emulsion. These organisms may lead to diagnosis of pyelonephritis, cystitis or pyometra. They may be in chains of streptococci, etc.
5. *Parasitic eggs* are rare but often seen in urine of deshi pigs due to *Stephanurus dentatus* infection (common in India), capillaria, and *Dirofilaria immitis* infection.

■ PRACTICAL KIDNEY ASSOCIATED CONDITIONS

Pulpy Kidney Disease

Pulpy kidney disease is produced by the toxins of *Clostridium perfringens* type D. The toxin is produced in the intestine after sudden change to rich food or due to feeding after long withdrawal of food. I observed that a flock of our sheep and goats was being tested for JD. After several hours, the animals got lush green sorghum with sorghum seeds. Next day, a large number of them were lying dead or lying with convulsions, groaning, opisthotonos, and semifluid faeces with mucous.

A smear from faeces stained by simple 1% methylene blue (after fixation with alcohol or spirit) revealed almost pure culture of bacilli under oil emersion microscopy. Urine of some animals gave positive test for glucose.

Management: I adopted intraperitoneal injection of intalyte mixed with cow colostral globulin (about 100–200 ml). Intaceph tazo was administered to control bacterial multiplication in intestine. Tonophosphan along with dextrose or intalyte was injected IP to revive energy and to treat hypothermia/negative energy balance. This intraperitoneal injection can be repeated after 1–2 hours. KOL or KOL L of Carus Laboratoris can be given orally. It absorbs the toxin.

Urinary Calculi (Stones)

Urinary calculi may form anywhere in the urinary organs such as in the kidney tissue, pelvis, ureter or urinary bladder. Urinary stones are more common in bullocks and camels.

Types: In cattle, stone are made of calcium carbonate, calcium phosphate and magnesium carbonate.

Vitamin A deficiency, lack of water (as in camels) and use of hard water helps in increase in cases of calculi.

Places where stones form:

Bullock and camel: Sigmoid flexure are 'S'-shaped curvature which passes a few inches below the anus and deep under the skin (Fig. 12.1).

Sheep and goats: Urethral end

Dogs: Above prostate gland and at the end of penis (os penis)

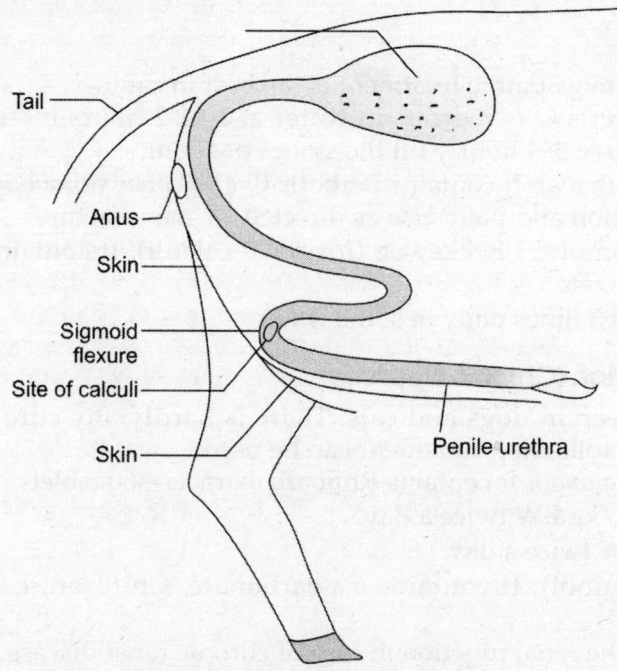

Fig. 12.1: S-shaped curvature

Symptoms

1. Uneasiness due to pain.
2. Sometimes blood in urine (haematuria) due to injury by stones.
3. Dribbling of urine in drops due to obstruction.
4. Stoppage of urine due to obstruction of urethra.
5. Urea level of blood may go up if micturation is obstructed.
6. Urinary bladder may rupture discharging urine into peritoneum and fatal uraemia may result.
7. Dogs cry due to pain and may vomit due to uraemia.

Diagnosis

1. From symptoms (stoppage or dribbling of urine.
2. Blood mixed urine.
3. X-ray examination.

Treatment

1. *Urethrectomy:* Cutting open at the sigmoid flexure in case of bullocks is a good surgical method.
2. Note pH of urine and give alkaline fluid orally if urine is acidic and acidic water if urine is alkaline.
3. Lyotaz injection (containing Piperacillin + Tazobactum) 4.5 g injection vial is dissolved in diluents (10 ml) and it treats the infection if any, and helps in release of calculus.
4. With the help of a catheter, push up normal saline into urethra slowly and steadily to flush out the stone.

Homoeopathic

In my experience, homoeopathic treatment is the best in canines.
1. Administer Berberis Q 6–7 drops in water at 1 or 2 hours intervals for about 4–5 times. Then give 3–4 hourly till the stones pass out.
2. Urisis drops (Lormans): It contains Berberis Q and other homoeopathic drugs to relieve inflammation and pain. Use as directed by manufacturer.
3. R-27 Combination of Dr Reckeweg (for renal calculi). It contains Berberis D3, Acidum Nitricum, etc.
   Dose: 10–15 drops 3 times daily in some water.

Chronic Renal Function (Chronic Nephritis)

This is sometimes seen in dogs and cats. There is hardly any cure for this but to prolong survival the following treatment can be used:
1. *Rubenal 300 (Vetoquinol):* It contains Rhubarb extracts—60 tablets
   Dose: Dog: 15 mg/kg BW twice a day.
   Cat: 25 mg/kg BW twice a day.
2. *Ipakitine* (Vetoquinol): It contains Ca carbonate, Chitosan, Lactose and Soy hydrolysate.
   Use: To support the renal function in case of chronic renal disease.
3. *Homoeopathic*: Rinakoll (Medisynth) syrup contains Berberis Q, Sarsaparilla, Tribulus terrestris, Chimaphila, Helonias, Dioica, Juniperus, and Vesicaria as Q potency.
   Dose: 1/2 teaspoonful twice a day.
   Small dog: 5–8 drops twice a day, for prevention of chronic recurrent urinary problems.

Pyelonephritis

Contagious bovine pyelonephritis is caused by *Corynebacterium renale* in cattle and occasionally in sheep. It may spread venerially or by catheter in mature cows.

Clinical picture: In summary, urine mixed with blood (haematuria), pus (pyuria) may occur along with colic and loss of condition. Urine pH is alkaline above 8. Direct microscopic examination of stained smears from exudates may show pleomorphic gram-positive bacterial rods.

Treatment: Large doses of procain penicillin (15000 IU/kg BW) may be injected daily for 3 weeks. Penicillin G procaine fortified by Zydus is best for treating *C renale* as well as calf diphtheria caused by corynebacteria in calves. Ceftriaxone and salbectum sodium injection (active agains G+ and G- bacteria) is a widespectrum injection (Celtrivan), available as 3 g vial. Inject about 10 mg/kg/ IM or IV. Repeat for 3–4 days.

Urinary Tract Infection (UTI)

Treatment: Marbomel and Marbofloxacin (Neovet)

Dose: 2–5 mg per kg BW once a day

Packing: strip of 5 tablets of 50 mg.

Enrodac (Zydus): Vial of 15 and 100 ml, 100 mg per ml. Inject 1 ml per 20 kg BW for 3–5 days.

■ CYSTITIS

Cystitis or inflammation of urinary bladder is almost similar to pyelonephritis regarding urinary findings and also the treatment. The only difference is dysuria which means painful urination which is more frequent and in small quantities. Presence of 1000 to 40,000 colony forming units of bacteria (CRU) per ml of urine strongly indicates bacterial cystitis.

Jackshot (Carus Lab, Karnal) stops haematuria due to cystitis or pyelonephritis. Injection: IM/IV and topical at the rate of 20 ml per large animal (450 kg) can be repeated 2–3 times a day for 2–8 days. It contains Tranexamic acid. For treating bacterial infection drugs mentioned under pyelonephritis may be used. Best are Oxytetracyclin L.A. of Zydus, Vetazo (Ceftriaxone + Tazobactam) of Zydus.

Cattle—dose is 5–10 mg/kg BW by IM/IV.

Dogs— 15–20 mg/kg BW by IM/IV.

■ HAEMATURIA

Haematuria is not a disease but a symptom seen due to several causes. Presence of blood in urine may be so small that urine may just look smoky but on test for blood by Benzidine, a clear positive result is seen. Causes of haematuria include cystitis, pyelonephritis, polypoid, cystitis in dogs, fungal (Aspergillus or Candida) infection after long antibiotic therapy, tumours of bladder or babesiosis in cattle.

■ ENZOOTIC HAEMATURIA

Enzootic haematuria of cattle is a specific disease of cattle seen mostly in hilly, unfertile soils where bracken ferns grow and are eaten by cattle with or without haemorrhagic cystitis or formation of haemangiomas in urinary bladder.

Treatment

1. Inject Jackshot as given above.
2. Inject Adchrome (G Leukatos Co) injection 5 ml per large animal IM for a few days particularly for blood in milk. Jackshot injection may also help in haemangiomas.
3. Give homoeopathic medicine Phosphorus 200 two teaspoonful 3–4 times a day by mouth. Thuza 1000, 30 drops daily may also be given if haemangioma is suspected.

■ HAEMOGLOBINURIA

Postparturient haemoglobinuria is most important. It is seen in hight milker cows and buffaloes. It is seen usually 2–4 weeks postcalving. It is more common in buffaloes in which local people use the term 'Lahoo moctan'.

Cause: Phosphorus deficiency due to following factors:
1. Too much feeding of cauliflower, alfa-alfa, etc.
2. Deficiency of phosphorus in soil or famines.
3. Draining out of phosphorus in colostrums in high milkers.

Symptoms: Light red or brown urine in mild cases and distinct red in severe. Drop in milk yield, dullness, fast breathing due to less oxygen in blood. Cool ears, tail, teats. Sometimes, gangrene in tail and ears. Heart rate goes up and is audible and strong. There is dehydration and dry constipated faeces. If untreated, the animal dies in 3 to 5 days due to ketosis. Body temperature drops below normal in late stages.

Diagnosis: Haemoglobinuria in high milkers, 2–3 weeks after parturition is the most important point to rul-out other causes.

Other causes of haemoglobinuria are babesiosis, bacillary haemoglobinuria due to *Clostridium haemolyticum* and leptospirosis in which fever is an important point to rule out as compared to hypothermia in postparturient haemoglobinuria in which fever is not seen.

Treatment:
1. T Phos injection (Zydus) 2 methy phenyl-phosphoric acid
   Acute large animal: 5–25 ml
   Small animal: 1–3 ml
   Give 50% dose IV and rest by SC or IM route at several sites. Repeat at few hours till improvement (Packing of 30 ml and 100 ml).
   Chronic cases: Postparturient paeresis: T. phos as above + Neuroxin M injection (Methy cobalamin injection)
   Small animals (chronic): 1–2 ml SC or IM daily
2. *Phosphovet Forte* (Merial): Butaphosphan + Cyanocobalamin injection) IM/IV
   10–25 ml; 5–12 ml, 2.5–5 ml per 30 kg BW.
3. *Metstorm*: Organic phosphorus + B_{12}
   Butaphosphan—100 mg/ml
   Cyanocobalamin—50 mcg/ml
   Cattle, horse, camel—10–25 ml by IV, IM, SC injection
   Calf/foal—5–12 ml by IV, IM, SC injection
   Sheep/goat—2.5–8 ml by IV, IM, SC injection
   Dog—0.5–5 ml by IV, IM, SC injection
4. *Tonolon injection* (Vets Pharma): Toldim phos sodium
   Indications: Haemoglobinuria, milk fever, vaginal or uterine prolaps
   Dose:
   Acute: 1 ml/20 kg BW
   Chronic: 1 ml/40 kg BW 1/2 dose by IV and 1/2 by IM or SC
5. *Bovirum bolus* (iron, Ant, Cu, Cobalt): Cattle and buffalo: 3–4 boli/day

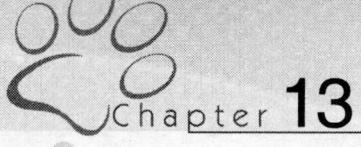

Chapter 13

Important Mineral Deficiency Diseases

■ HYPOMAGNESEMIC TETANY (GRASS TETANY, LACTATION TETANY)

Low body and blood magnesium leads to hyperaesthesia and muscular excitement, leading to incoordination during walking, tetanus like spasms and convulsions.

Etiology and Pathogenesis

1. Too much feeding of grass, particularly fresh crop which is low in magnesium.
2. *Lactation tetany*: Mostly seen in mares, occasionally in cows, which have high milk yield and which get too much green grass.
3. In calves of 2–4 months age it is more common if fed on whole milk. Normal serum magnesium of calves is 2–2.25 mg/dl. In tetany it is around 0.6 mg/dl.

Symptoms

Hypersensitivity of muscles, excessive movement of ears, spasms on touching the body, opisthotonos, kicking under the belly, champing of jaws, stamping of feet, etc. Pulse rate goes up to 200–250/minute in terminal stages. Death in a short-time after weak pulse and cyanosis (bluing of mucosa).

Treatment

Injection of 100 ml of 10% solution of magnesium sulphate may provide day-to-day relief. For long-term treatment to replenish bone reserve, magnesium oxide may be given orally at the rate of 1 g/day for 10 days for calves under 5 weeks of age and 2 g for calves of 5–10 weeks age. Magnesium carbonate may be given as alternative in double dose. 'Magical ' injection of Cadila may be injected, available as 450 ml bottle. 'Mifex' milk fever formula can also be injected.

Preventive

1. *Minfa Active (Intas)*: 1 kg/100 kg feed contains copper, cobalt, magnesium, iron, zinc, and chromium (10 kg bag; cattle).
2. *Minfa F5 (Intas)*: 10 kg and 30 kg bags. Contents as for Minfa active + phosphorous, potassium, iodine, and sulphur.
   Dose: 1 kg in 100 kg feed (cattle).
3. *Petmina tablets*: Contain chelated minerals, vitamins, amino acids, DHA and antioxidents (improves metabolism, health, skin problems, hairs, and old age problems). A Kepler product.
   Dose: For puppies 1/2 tab twice, Dogs: 1 tablet per day.
4. *Petspro powder (Kepler product)*: Probiotics, prebiotics, and minerals.
   Dose: For puppies, 2 g TDS; dogs (small)—4 g TDS; 8 g (large dogs).

5. *VM 365 (MSD product)*: Same as Petmina.
6. *VM-P (MSD product)*: All 16 minerals + vitamins A, D_3, E, K. Available as 5 kg, 25 kg bags.
   Dose: Cows—100–200 g/10 kg feed; calf 25–30 g/day; sheep/goat 15–20 g/day.
7. *Vitamix Gold (Zydus)*: Maximum Biotin (Vitamin H), udder health; liquid 60 ml and 300 ml packs: vitamins A, D_3, E, B_{12}, biotin, energy.
   Dose: 10 ml daily for cows; calves 5 ml daily.
8. *Lactiphos injection (Eldin Pharma):* Phosphonic acid salt for postparturient haemeglobinuria, low milk, hypophosphatemia and infertility. 30 ml vial.
   Dose: Cattle and buffaloes 10–15 ml; small animals 1–3 ml IM, IV, SC injection.
9. *Tinaphos:* Injection (Tineta Pharma), 30 ml vial; dose as for lactiphos.
10. Tonophosphan (MSD, Intervet India): vials of 10 and 30 ml.
    Dose as for Lactiphos.
11. *Other products are:*
    Catasol (Bayer) 15 ml vials; dose 1 ml per 33 kg BW for 3–5 days.
    Urimin (Virbac): Sodium acid phosphate injection; 10 and 30 ml vial.
    Dose: cattle 10–15 ml; calves 1–3 ml; dogs 1–2 ml IM, IV, SC.

■ COPPER DEFICIENCY

Nowadays, due to green revolution, mineral imbalance of copper is becoming more common. It may be of two types:
1. *Primary:* Due to soil deficiency, hence plant deficiency in sandy soils, more in spring and summer.
2. *Secondary:* High molybdenum or sulphur in plants retards copper absorption by plants/fodder.
   Copper can be given as preventive or curative ingredient. I have used copper injections with good results.

Disease/signs: 10 to 20 mg copper/kg of dry matter is toxic. Deficiency is endemic, all over the world but it goes undetected because of slow symptoms and poor knowledge of veterinarians. In UK about 9% of cattle, particularly heifers, show Cu deficiency.

Types: a. *"Enzootic ataxia"*: Sudden weakness, leading mainly to weakness of hind quarters, animal (calf) may assume sitting posture, growth is poor, tendency for diarrhoea, paresis, incoordination, fracture of limbs. Skin coat itching, loss of normal colour of hairs since copper is necessary for skin pigment (depigmentation). In terminal stages, the animal falls suddenly on side, bellows, and dies due to heart failure. Loss of hair pigment is best seen around the eyes, giving 'spectacled appearance'.

Goats and lambs: The disease is called "Sway back". Newborn are born weak or dead; paralysis of hind legs is of spastic type. Cerebral white matter is poorly developed.

Prevention

1. *Minfa (Active)*—as suggested above
2. *Minfa FS*—as suggested above

I prescribe a pinch of Ferrous sulphate (560 mg) + copper sulphate (120 mg) + zinc sulphate (300 mg) in calf starter daily during growing age. Periodical monitoring of haemoglobin and if anaemia is significant, then following injections:

1. *Minfa shot (Intas product):* Injection in 10 and 50 ml vials; contains zinc, manganese, copper and selenium
   Dose: Cows/buffaloes up to 1 year age 1 ml/50 kg BW; 1–2 years 1 ml/35 kg SC or IM
2. *Feritas bolus* (Fe + folic acid + B_{12}) strips of 5 boli
   Dose: 2 boli daily for 10–15 days
3. *Feritas injection (Intas)*: Dose 1 ml /50 kg BW, IM in 3 days till normal haemoglobin develops (10–20 days)
4. *Micro powder (Neospark):* 250 ml and 1 litre. 10 ml = 15000 mcg Cu; 9000 mcg Co 6000 mcg Selenium; 15000 mcg Zn
   Cow: 15–30 ml/day
   Calf: 5–10 ml/day
5. *Vets Cu Co* (Vets Pharma Ltd, www.vetsfarma.com): It contains copper and cobalt in tablet form.
   Dose: Cattle: 4 tabs daily for 2–3 weeks; sheep, goat, calves: 2 tabs daily for 2–3 weeks
6. *Rumen FS (Alembic):* Bolus of iron, Cu, Co, B_1, B_{12}, yeast.
   Dose: 2 boli twice daily for 5 days.

■ COBALT DEFICIENCY

This deficiency occurs in ruminants. Actually, it is B_{12} deficiency. In cattle, the disease is named 'Enzootic marasmus' or 'Wasting disease'.

I have observed cobalt and copper deficiency on mass scale in cattle, sheep, and goats of Surat Panjrapole where I work as Consultant Veterinarian. I use Copper oxide and Cobaltous chloride hexahydrate in my own formulation of injections which very well control 'Falling disease' (Cu deficiency) and 'Enzootic marasmus' (Cobalt deficiency) promptly. The disease is more common in spring when Cobalt (and Cu) absorption cannot keep pace with fast grown (fertilizer promoted) grass, sorghum, maize, etc. to absorb adequate cobalt. Like copper deficiency, cobalt deficiency also may be of two types:

1. Primary—deficiency in soil, more common.
2. Secondary—due to imbalance of other minerals.

Symptoms

The most important guiding points to suspect cobalt deficiency are:

1. Loss of BW (marasmus).
2. Loss of appetite.
3. Pica (tendency to eat abnormal things, bones, plastic, etc.).
4. Anaemia (pale conjunctivae) and fatigue.
5. Too much lacrimation (tears) and nasal discharge (important).
6. Symptoms most severe at 6 months age; death in 3–12 months.
7. 'White liver' in sheep at postmortem or slaughter; 'fatty liver' in goats.

■ MANAGEMENT OF COBALT DEFICIENCY

Prevention

1. *Minotas (Bovicura/Intas):* contains copper, cobalt, zinc, manganese, selenium, iodine, vitamins A and E. Packing in strip of 7 boli. Dose: 1 bolus alternate days for 7 days.
2. *Minshot (Bovicura, Intas):* All above minerals in injectable form (10 ml and 50 ml). Adult cows and buffaloes below 1 year; Dose—1 ml/50 kg BW; above 1 year 1 ml/75 kg BW.
3. *Minotas-AV (Intas Aviglo):* Contains iron, Cu, Co, chromium, selenium, iodine, zinc, and manganese to prevent mineral deficiency; 25 kg bag. Dose: 1 kg/tonne feed.
4. *Provical Fort (Cargil),* Provimi A. Nautr. Pvt Ltd, Bangaluru): Ca, Ph, Zn, Cu, Co, iodine, vitamin D_3 and B_{12}. Dose: Cow/ buffalo; 10 ml/day (1, 5, 10, 20 litre packs).
5. *VM-P (MSD,* Intervet India Pvt Ltd): 25 kg pack. Mix ture as above. Dose: cow/ buffalo: 25–30 g /head/day; sheep and goats: 15–20 g/head/day.
6. *Minal Forte (Alembic):* Like provical but also contains lysine, methionine, fluorine (pack of 1 kg and 10 kg powder). Dose: 28 g/day/cow or buffalo.
7. *PHIL powder (Tineta Pharma Pvt Ltd):* Mixture as of above-mentioned minerals, pack of 1, 2.5, and 10 kg.
8. *Lykamin Fort (Lyka):* Like provical fort. Pack of 1 kg and 10 kg. Dose: Large animals—30 g/day; small animals 15 g/day.

Treatment

To my knowledge, there is no preparation to treat Cu and Co deficiency but Radostis et al 2000, Vety med 9th edition have mentioned 0.1 to 3 mg (oral) per day for calf. I have used cobaltous chloride hexahydrate, extra pur to prepare injections by dissolving in Belamy and Nuroxin M. to contain 2 mg of cobaltous chloride (beware: it is toxic above a limit) and inject 2 mg cobalt/day to be repeated after 7 days till recovery with good results. (Obtained from HiMedia laboratories Pvt Ltd, Mumbai).

■ PICA

Pica means depraved appetite in which condition animals, mostly cattle, start eating abnormal items such as:
1. Eating dung/faeces (coprophagia).
2. Bones (osteophagia).
3. Soil (geophagia).
4. Hairs of self or other animals (pitophagia).
5. Plastic, paper, iron pieces, etc.

Etiology

Phosphorus deficiency is strongly suspected but it is not the only cause. Presence of parasites and imbalanced and poor food can also contribute to it. Eating plastic bags is a great menace in India.

Treatment

See under phosphorus deficiency.

▪ PHOSPHORUS DEFICIENCY

Phosphorus deficiency is usually primary and the main guiding symptoms are listed below:

1. Poor growth in all species leading to rickets.
2. Pica-eating abnormal items like bone (see previous chapter for pica).
3. Osteodystrophia (softening of bones).
4. Lethargy and fractures.
5. Infertility after months of deficiency (in cows).
6. Stiffness in forelegs in cattle ('*Creaps*' or '*peg legs*').
7. Haemoglobinuria in high-milk yielding cows. Mostly red soil areas are deficient in phosphorus.
8. Arching back and stiff gait.
   80–85% of phosphorus of body is located in bones.

Diagnosis

Blood P levels falls down 1.3 to 1.7 from the normal of 4–5 mg/L.
Serum Ca levels are usually unaffected.

Prevention and Treatment

Dietary P of 0.38 to 0.40% is enough for high yielding cows.

Example:

1. *Cal Shakti Platina* (Bovicura/Intas) 1 litre and 5 litres packs
   Dose: Heavy milkers—50 ml twice a day
   Non-milkers—25 ml twice a day
   Calves—20 ml twice a day
   Sheep/goats—5 ml twice a day
2. *Ultra Phos* (Neospark)—Sodium acid phosphate injections
   Large animals —7.5–10 ml
   Small animals—2.5–5 ml IM, IV, or SC
3. *Calcium Best Granules* (—Ca, P, and all other trace minerals (Brovet Animal Health Care, Navsari, Gujarat), also Chelated Magical DS—oral liquid
4. *INO Milk (Hester Biosciences, Ahmedabad):* Ca and P, oral—Cattle 50 ml B/D
   Calves—25 ml B/D
5. *Phosphovet Forte (Merial):* Injection of 30 ml and 90 ml contains butaphosphan and cyanocobalamin for postparturient haemoglobinuria, infertility, pica, anoestrus.
   Dose: Cattle, buffalo, horse: 10–25 ml; calf/foal: 5–12 ml; sheep/goat 2.5–5 ml IM or IV Repeat daily till recovery.
6. Lactophos injections (Eldin pharma)
   Dose: 10–15 ml for large animals
   1–3 ml for small animals
7. *Soda Phos* (Zydus, powder, 500 g packing)
   Dose: 60–100 g daily for 5 to 10 days for reduced fertility, pica, haematuria, arched back.

Other:
1. General cases 'Metabolin' injection (Hester product, Hester Biosciences, Ahmedabad): It contains butaphosphan 100 mg, cyanocobalamin 50 mcg.
   Dose: Cattle 10--25 ml; calf 5–12 ml; sheep/goat 2.5–8 ml IV/IM/SC routes on every 3 days till recovery.
2. *Lykamin Forte (Lyka product):* Contains all essential minerals including Ca and P. Feed regularly to large animals 30 g daily; small animals 15 g daily (packing of 1 kg and 10 kg).
3. *Tonegil (Toldimfos Sodium injction):* It is a sterile, clear and stable solution for parenteral administration of Toldimfos Sodium. It is a good nontoxic phosphorous preparation for the regulation of metabolic process. It acts not only on skeletal muscles, but also stimulates smooth muscles such as uterus, bladder, etc. and has a toning action on the myocardium. Good for growth of calves, bones, reduction of convalescence period, pregnancy, regular milk production, anoestrus condition, metabolic diseases, debility emaciation, and pica too.
   Dose: Large animals—15 ml as regularly as possible; 20 ml for 2–3 days in post-parturient Haemoglobinuria.
   Small animals: 1–3 ml, half the dose by *intravenous route* and *half by intramuscular or subcutaneous route.*
   Packs: Vials of 10 ml and 30 ml.

■ CALCIUM DEFICIENCY: RICKETS AND OSTOMALACIA

Rickets

It is due to calcium deficiency in all growing animal species, characterised by misshapen bones, deformed legs (bowing of legs), lameness and stiffness. Most common in pups.

Osteomalacia

Calcium deficiency in adult animals, mainly cows results in weak, porous bones resulting in lordosis (concave vetetebral column).

Rich sources of calcium are bone meal (powder), lime stone, legumes, forages (1.42%).

There are large number of calcium additives which are regularly provided to valuable animals at dose recommended by manufacturer. Such mixtures also contain phosphorus, copper, cobalt, chromium, vitamins, mainly vitamin D_3, etc. Examples are:
1. *Capsola Gold:* Chelated double power. It contisns Ca, P, D_3, Cu, B_{12}, Mn, Zn, shatavari and Jivanti. Helpful in maximising milk production.
2. *Caldisol-DC Solution*: It contains Ca gluconate, Cu D saccharate, ferric ammon. Citrate, gluconate, and B_{12}. It is used in high milkers, pregnancy, and in lactating animals.
   Cows, etc. 50 ml twice a day.
   Calf, sheep, goats, pigs, foals: 20 ml, twice a day
   Dose: 10 ml twice a day, orally.
   It is a very good, crystal clear solution.
3. *Vetcal B_{12}* (Zydus): Flavoured syrup.

Contents: Ca. phosphate $Ca_3 (PO_4)_2$, cholecalciferol (vitamin D), B_{12} in flavoured suspension.

Use: milk yield, rickets, osteomalacia, milk fever, pregnancy, poor growth, Pica.

Dose: Cows, etc. 100 ml twice a day

Calf 20 ml twice a day

Dog 10 ml twice a day

Packing 500 ml and 5 litres

4. *Supplevite-M*: contents: Vitamins A, D_3, B_{12}, E, K, choline, Ca, Mg, iodine, iron, zinc, Cu, Co.

Add 1 kg in 400 kg feed

5. *Supplevite-M Gold* (Zydus): It contains all the above minerals plus selenium, potassium, sodium, sulphur, nicotinamide, iodine, and chromium.

Dose: Cow, etc. 30 g/day (normal)

Milkers and horses: 50 g/day

Calf, sheep, goat, pig: 15 g/day

6. *Cadisol DC solution* (Zydus): Contains Ca, D saccharate, B_{12}, iron in crystal clear solution.

Dose: 50 ml twice daily for cows and buffaloes

20 ml twice daily for calves, sheep and goats; 10 ml twice daily for dogs

Packing: 100, 500 ml and 1 and 5 litres

7. *Vetcal B_{12} (Zydus)*: 500 ml and 5 litres containers.

8. *Vetcal Gold B_{12} (Zydus):* Cows, etc. 100 ml/day

Goat, pigs, etc. 20 ml, twice a day

9. *Ascal Gold*: Chelated (Alembic)

Similar to Vetcal + Shatavari, Biotin and Javitri

Dose: Cows, etc. in milk: 100 ml twice a day

10. *Minal Forte*: Minerals + amino acids, lysine, methionine, fluorine in flavoured syrup. Useful as no 9 above.

Powder: Dose 10 g/day for cows

Packing: 1 kg and 10 kg.

11. *Caldhan V (Dabur)*: Solution form containing Ca, Phos, D_3, B_{12}

Dose: Cow, etc. 50 ml; calves, etc. 20 ml; goat, etc. 10 ml

12. *Holler* (Kepler product): Contains Ca, P, Zn, Cu, Co, Fe, Sel., D_3, A, E.

Packing: 10 boli, Dose: Cow, etc. 2 boli

13. *VM powder* (MSD product): A very good product containing all minerals and vitamins, A, D, E, K.

14. *VM-P powder (MSD)*: As above + Biotin 2% and chromium.

Dose as for VM powder

15. *Vibra Cal Gel* (Neospark): Contains Ca, P and other minerals in gel form. 250 g available as oral tube.

Use: 1 tube 12 hours postcalving. Repeat at 12 hours till necessary. It is palatable and easily eaten by cow.

16. *Inomilk Gold*: Suspension 5 litres. Contains Ca, P, B_{12}, Biotin, Jeevanti, Satavari.

Dose: Cow, etc. (in milk): 50 ml BID orally.

17. *Merical Pet (Vetoquinol product):* Briswuits. Contains Ca, P, D_3, and B_{12} in 5 litre jars.

Dose: Dogs, etc. 1–2 brisquits/day; cats, etc. 1/2 brisquit/day

18. *Calup Gel (Cargil product):* This is available as a plastic collapsible tube each containing 43.5 g ionic (Ca) for prevention and safety against milk fever. Give one tube gel before and 1 tube gel after parturition.

19. *Balanion powder (Zydus):* Blend of anionic Ca, P.

    Indications: As for Calup gel above.

    Dose: 50 g (one packet) daily for 10 days before parturition and 10 days daily postparturition (1 box of 20 packets)

    Other products of calcium are: Calshakti DS 2.5 litres; Calboral injection 450 ml (Novartis); Caldhan liquid 5 litres (Dabur), Mifex injection (450 ml (Novartis), Mifex oral 1 and 5 litres.

■ CALCIUM DEFICIENCY

Cows require 31 g calcium daily during pregnancy for foetal requirements and maintenance of self. In late gestation period, 100 g Ca/day for cow can be provided easily by normal diet. In dry period, 10–12 g/day is required. Due to calving, the normal dietary Ca falls short suddenly, leading to hypocalcaemia. Prepartum feed high in phosphorus (80 g/day) also results in hypocalcaemia and milk fever, as also by high sodium and potassium cations (legumes).

Milk Fever (Parturient Paresis—Downer Cow Syndrome)

Hosts: Cattle, sheep, and goats. Mature animals, usually 5–10 years old and rare in 1st and 2nd calvings. Jerseys are most susceptible as also some Indian breeds (high milkers).

Time: Milk fever occurs in three stages:
 1. Past few days of pregnancy.
 2. Most common—48 hours after calving, up to the tenth day.
 3. Few weeks before calving.

■ IODINE DEFICIENCY

Iodine deficiency leads to:
 1. Reproductive failure with abnormally developed organs, failure to return to estrus or suppressed estrus, silent heat, failure to zygote formation, arrested foetal development, early embryonic death, failure to nidate implant, conception failure, abortions, repeat breeding, dystokia-abnormal parturition, uterine prolapse, retention of placenta, infertility, stillbirth, and prolonged gestation period.
 2. In males, poor fertility, poor libido, poor semen quality, low quantity of semen, and poor mating efficiency.
 3. It can also lead to poor growth, and unthriftiness.
 4. In terms of production, to poor milk yield, higher incidence of ketosis, delayed peak lactation, shorter lactation period, and sometimes, failure in letting down or delayed letting down of milk.
 5. In terms of udder development, poorly developed udder, variable teat size, leaky teats, non-functioning teats, and hard texture of teats.

6. Problems related to thermoregulation such as subnormal body temperature, high temperature in hot season and in high humid weather, poor heat resistance or heat intolerance syndrome, and panting.
7. Anorexia and poor metabolism lead to overall weak animal. Apart from this, the animal may fall sick often due to poor resistance and low immunity caused by lack of iodine.

Treatment

1. 'Iodised salt' used to be the safest and most practical means of providing supplementary dietary iodine.
2. Other sources include calcium iodate, cuprous iodide, and calcium.
3. *Elemental iodine injection:* I-Fer-H is elemental iodine for parenteral administration and it provides prompt response and immediate action. It is composed of elemental iodine 150 mg/ml.

   Indications: To control fibrous tissue formation in mastitis, hypothermia, hyperthermia in heat intolerance, actinobacillosis, actinomycosis.

   Administration is to be via subcutaneours or intramuscular injection.
4. *V-5 injection is another* good product which provides elemental iodine with four vitamins, viz. vitamin A, D, E, and biotin. It produces synergistic action on squamous and sphincter muscle cells as well as other endocrine glands. Vitamin E acts as antioxidant and vitamins A and D help in terms of metabolism, haematopoiesis, antioxidant activity, etc. thereby enhancing immunity and endocrine functions apart form the benefits of iodine.

   Composition: Each 5 ml vial contains iodine 750 mg, vitamin A 250000 IU, biotin 125 mcg, vitamin D 25000 IU, vitamin E 1001 IU.

   Indications: To control fibrous tissue formation in mastitis, hypothermia, heat intolerance syndrome, actinobacillosis, actinomycosis, poor developed udder, non-functioning teat on postmastitis, leaky teats, dissimilar teat size, and to combat transport stress.

   Presentation: 5 ml, 10 ml vials with disposable syringe.

   Dose: 1 ml/80 kg BW may be repeated after 3 months according to requirements.

   Administration: IM or SC.

Chapter 14

Important Toxic Conditions

■ CHRONIC SELENOSIS (BLIND STAGGERS, ALKALI DISEASE)

Selenium is essential for metabolism of proteins (selanoproteins) and enzymes (selanoenzymes). It is in excess quantity in some geographical areas such as Punjab, Haryana and is more aggravated by winter.

Symptoms

1. Progressive emaciation and rough body coat.
2. Overgrowth (long) of hooves with horizontal cracks and lameness.
3. Loss of appetite, delayed oestrus.
4. Gangrene, followed by sloughing of tail.
5. Blood picture is normal.
6. Stiff gait or lameness.

Control

Right concentration of selenium in the ruminants is 0.1 to 1.0 mg/kg of feed. Higher selenium containing soils are called selanophorous areas. The top 60–90 cm of soil contains maximum selenium. Selenium should not be more than 5 mg/kg of dry feed. To tontrol selenium toxicity in pigs, 0.01–0.02% arsanilic acid or 0.005% of 3 nitro 4 hydroxyphenyl arsenic acid in ration or 550 mg/day to growing cattle gives some protection along with high protein diet. A single oral dose of 20–40 mg/kg of copper given 24 hours prior to toxic selenium is reported to antagonise selenium. In cattle, 0.01 arsanilic acid in diet may give slight protection. Adding linseed oil in ration improves protection against selenium toxicity.

■ NITRATE-NITRITE TOXICITY

I have observed this problem several times which probably goes unreported or undiagnosed. The main causes of poisoing are given below:

1. *Excessive use of nitrogenous fertilizers associated with low rainfall/irrigation* leads to accumulation of nitrates in the stems of fast growing seasonal crops like maize, sorghum, etc.
2. *Seepage of nitrates into soil of high fertilizer treated soils* into subsoil (tubewells) or well water.
3. *Effluents from meat establishments* where nitrates are used to preserve colour of meat, also whey making plants.
4. *Silage making* may result in more nitrates in the lower strata of silage pit.
5. *Contamination with nitrogenous fertilizers such as urea.*
6. *In areas where hard water contains 2300 ppm of nitrate may be toxic.*

Susceptibility

Pigs are more susceptible than cattle, sheep, and goats in that order. Poorly fed animals which suddenly get nitrate rich fodder are also susceptible.

Pathogenesis

The nitrates are broken down by rumen microflora (crores of bacteria and protozoa per ml) into nitrite or further, into ammonia. Ammonia itself is absorbed and goes to liver where the surplus ammonia in the blood is highly toxic to brain, resulting in recumbancy. Nitrites in blood form methaemoglobin, making colour of RBCs/blood to turn chocolate coloured. Methaemoglobin stops oxygen transport by RBCs hence there is hypoxia. This conversion may take a few hours to show clinical effects summarised below:

1. *Death, if 76–88%* of haemoglobin is converted into methaemoglobin.
2. Dyspnoea due to hypoxia, with gasping—animals may *breathe with open mouth* and protruding tongue, like dog.
3. *Cyanosis means bluish/dark colour of skin* and mucus membranes.
4. *Muscle tremors (twitching)* due to hypoxia and stumbling gait.
5. *Tachycardia and subnormal body temperature.*
6. *Abortion.*
7. Chocolate coloured blood.

Diagnosis

1. *Diphenylamine test*: This is a simple test for which the reagent can be kept without expiry for years. The reagent is prepared as below:
   - 0.5% diphenylamine
   - 20 ml distilled water
   Add concentrated sulphuric acid to make 100 ml.
   The suspected plant (inside of stem) is dipped in the above solution. If intense blue clolur develops in the stem, it indicates more than 1% nitrate in the plant. The same method I have used by adding the solution as a layer on clotted blood or aqueous humour or urine. Blue colour develops in positive case by slowly adding the above reagent (even from dead animal).
2. *Commercial test strips*: I use a very simple test strip to test liquid from plants, drinking water, serum, etc. with quantitative results.
   I use Quantofix (nitrate nitrite) test strips to get quantity mg/L NO_3 as 10, 25, 50, 100, 200, and 500 (mg/L) within a few seconds after wetting or dipping in the plant fluid, water urine, aqueous humour and serum.
   Manufacturers are Macherey-Nagel, Neumann-Neanderstr, 6-8-52355 Duran, Germany. One packet contains about 100 test strips which give reliable results even for 2 years postexpiry by experimental proof (by dipping in solutions of sodium nitrate).
   Nitrate nitrite: Toxicity
   Semiquantitative test papers for following toxic chemicals are also available as test papers (Qualigens fine chemicals)
   Code M1304—Copper—0–10, 30, 100, 300 ppm
   Code M1318—Cyanide—0–1, 3: 10, 30, ppm

Code M 1325—Molybdenum—0, 5, 20, 50, 100, 250 ppm
Code M 1313 Nitrate 0, 10, 25, 50, 100, 250, 500 ppm
Nitrite 0, 1, 5, 10, 20, 40, 80 ppm

Prevention and Control

Methylene blue is specific antidote of methaemoglobin which converts methaemoglobin to haemoglobin. 1 to 2 mg/kg BW is injected as 1% solution IV. In ruminants, 20 mg/kg BW can be used. Methylene blue powder is available (25 g pack) from RFCL, RANKEM, A3, Industrial Area, Okhla, Phase I, New Delhi 110020.

Ascorbic Acid injections (5 ml) are produced by Juggat Pharma at cheap rate of ₹ 3.92/5 ml. This can also be injected for relief from nitrate toxicity (SC or IM injection).

As preventive, the green fodder (mature) should be cautiously switched over, preferably after diphenylamin test which takes a few seconds and is least expensive. The solution remains stable for years (I used it for 6 years). Stop suspected grass or silage immediately. Sometimes, nitrate nitrite fertilisers accidentally added to food may cause toxicity.

▓ AFLATOXICOSIS

Aflatoxin is a fungal toxin produced by *Aspergillus flavus* and some other Aspergillus species. Most important is groundnut cake or maize but any other food item can be toxic too if its moisture content is above 10%. Such feed mixtures are hot if hand is introduced deep into it (heat generated by fungal growth).

Main Symptoms

Retardation of growth in calves, reduced milk yield, dullness, diarrhoeic feaces with or without blood and jaundice (if advanced), blindness and circling movements are observed. Ascites in dogs is common as also in poultry, particularly broilers.

Treatment

Mytox nil powder (Lyka): It contains toxin binding HSCAS and MOS and *Propionibacterium fruendenreichii* 50 billion CFU. It binds toxins and absorbs moisture in feed (1 kg pack).

Dose: Mix 1 kg/tonne feed (tested in Tamil Nadu Veterinary University).

Also give *Hepa Forte (Liver tonic)* containing choline, etc. Large animal 50 ml daily; small animal 10 ml daily.

▓ ENDOTOXINS

Endotoxins may be produced as a part of infections or fever.

1.

Name	Indications	Dose	Administration
Fluxivet injection, product of Carus Labs, New Delhi	Acute respiratory disease; acute coliform mastitis, fever, pain, diarrhoea, muscle skeletal disorder	2 ml/45 kg BW as IV or IM injection	Once a day or divided into two doses, given 12 hourly

Packing: 20, 50, and 100 ml.

2. *Vigest*: A general tonic and appetite stimulant. Contains polypeptide and short chain molecule dextrose and electrolytes.

   Use: Pour over feed mixture or mix with milk and feed orally.

   Dose: Cattle: 60–100 ml

   Calves, foals: 30–60 ml

   Sheep, goats, etc: 15–30 ml

   Dogs, cats: 2.5–5 ml

   Packing: 500 ml (Bayer Healthcare).

3. *Hepotas*: It is a combination of minerals, choline, vitamin E, and live yeast to protect and enhance liver function (25 kg bag). Add at the rate of 500 g to 1 kg/tonne of feed.

4. *Kol or Kol-L*: Please refer to drug index use of these drugs which contain activated charcoal which absorbs endotoxins from intestine to some extent.

Chapter 15

Diseases of Reproductive System and Mammary Glands in Ruminants

▣ RETENTION OF PLACENTA (ROP)

Placenta may not be cleared out after parturition. It may be accompanied by (a) sub-involution or without expulsion, (b) haemorrhage, (c) postpartum atony, (d) metritis and (e) pyometra. Expulsion up to 12 hours after delivery is considered normal.

Treatment

Ecbolics, generally herbal drugs act better than the allopathic medicines. See also the chapter on pyometra.

1. *Utripulse (Zydus)*: Contains about 16 herbal products. It cleans out easily, sets early onset of postpartum heat; it is safe, painless, and aseptic.
   Dose: Cow and buffaloes: 100–125 ml (orally)
         Mare: 50–75 ml
         Ewe, doe: 20–40 ml
   Give twice daily for 2–3 days after normal parturition. If ROP give 3 times dose every 3 hourly.

2. *Ergometrin injection* (Zydus): Contains methylergomatrine maleate 1 mg/ml
   Dose: Cow and buffaloes: 2–5 ml
   Ewe, doe: 0.5–1
   IM/IV Store at 2–8°C.

3. *Metricare (Intrauterine)*: It contains povidone iodine 5% w/v and metronidazole 1%
   It is destructive for most of the bacteria and prevents pyometra, cervicitis, and ROP.
   Introduce 30–60 ml intrauterine. Repeat at 24 hours interval for 2 more days.

4. *Proshe (Intas)*: It is a herbal product. It is administered orally at the rate of 100–125 ml twice and daily for 3–5 days.

5. *Oriprim 'U' bolus (Zydus)*: Place 2–4 boli in uterus after parturition. Repeat after 24 hours. (Presentation in 4 boli strip)
   Advantageous in preventing the above diseases.

6. *Exapar (Dabur Ayurvet Ltd)*: Contains 3 herbal ingredients
   Uses: ROP, poor reproduction, cotherapy pyometra. Presentation in 500 ml bottle and 4 boli blister pack. Give 4 boli orally twice daily and 2 boli twice for next 3 days. Or 100 ml liquid for 3 days twice a day.
   Besides this, it is better to give 500 ml of "Speedup" (of Natural Remedies) or Hyporid (Intas) 90 g twice daily. They contain ionic calcium.

7. *Himrop (Himalaya)*: It is available in liquid form in 500 ml bottle for placental expulsion.
   Dose: 100 ml twice a day, 1st day
   100 ml once a day × 3 days
8. *Metra*: 13 herbs make this liquid (Tineta Pharma, Powai, Mumbai 400072; phone: 022-28471611, 12)
   Dose: 75 to 100 ml daily orally (500 ml and 1 litre pack)
   Routine: Manual removal. Injection *Melonex* 30 ml—Belamyl Injection 10 ml—*Involon bolus* 3 + 3 morning and evening.

■ PROLAPSE OF UTERUS

Uterus and/or vagina may get prelapsed out of external genitalia. This may be habitual or spontaneous postpartum.

Treatment

1. To prevent threatened or habitual abortion *G Plex bolus* (Van Vet, Shalin Complex, Gandhinagar, Gujarat, phone: 9375046501; 16 bolus in 1 pack) Give 4 to 6 bolus twice daily.
2. Nexbolic (Neo Vet/Intas): Hastens uterine involution. Contains Methyl Ergometrine maleate 1 mg in 5 ml vial. Give IM/IV 2–5 mg in cattle, buffalo; 0.5–1 mg in sheep and goats within 24 hours postpartum.
3. *C flox TZ I'U.* (Neovet/Intas): Infuse 30 to 60 ml into uterus (packing of 60 ml. It is a broad-spectrum antibiotic.
4. *Inflavet injection*: Meloxicam with lignocaine and paracetamol injection. This stops straining and helps in pushing back (manually) prolapsed uterus. Dose: 2–3 ml per 33 kg BW IM/IV, SC route (presentation of 50 ml vial).
5. *Clinterus* (Kepler product): Kepler Vet Mission, Ahmedabad product. Contains 4 herbal products in a jar of 450 ml. It has dual function as potent ecbolic and for involution of prolapsed.
   Dose: Orally 100 ml for large animals × 3–5 days; 50 ml for small animals × 3–5 days.
6. *Epidosin*: Antispasmodic and painkiller. Helps in prolapsed reduction; Dose: Cattle 10–15 ml IM.
7. *Lignocain injection* 2% (Ecogen and Commo products): Inject 8–10 ml between tail berterrae to reduce spasms in uterus. This stops activity of nerves which produce expulsion.
8. *Siquil injection* may be used to sedate the animal during and after involution.
   Dose: Cow—10 mg IV or 20 mg IM (0.5 to 1 ml per 200 and 100 kg BW); Sheep—0.5 ml/100 kg BW.

■ MASTITIS

Mastitis is the most common and economically important disease of cows, sheep, goats, and other species. Most common causes are bacteria, viz:
1. *Streptococcus agalactiae, Staphylococcus aureus, Mycoplasma* species.
2. *Escherichia coli*—possibly with selenium and vitamin E deficiency. Take care for 2 weeks before calving and 2 weeks before dry spell (Fig. 15.1b).
3. Occasionally *Streptococcus uberis, Streptococcus dysgalactiae.*

4. Fungus: After too long use of antibiotics. *Cryptococcus necformans*, *Nocardia* sp., *Candida* species.

Gross Appearance

In acute stage, there is inflammation, swelling, stagnation of milk flow. In chronic stages, fibrosis and oedema develops. Usually more than one quarter of glands are affected. Flakes of clotted milk appear on milking. Later, the milk may become thick and pus-like.

Staphylococcal Mastitis

The symptoms vary between less pathogenic to highly pathogenic bacteria. In severe form there is redness, swelling and pain. It may get gangrenous with colour changing to blue-black and there is exudation of blood tinged fluid.

In less severe staphylococcal mastitis, the gland takes a course similar to streptococcal mastitis. Abscesses of variable size are scattered in the gland. Such form is seen usually after parturition.

Mycoplasmal Mastitis

This is caused in cows by *Myoplasma bovis*, *M. californicum* and *M. canadense*. Sometimes, otitis pneumonia and arthritis are observed in calves. It is highly contagious and spreads fast by milkers. In USA 1% iodine or betadine is used to externally to kill mycoplasma during an outbreak.

Milk becomes thin, watery like whey and may have a few white flakes. Or it may become thick like colostrum. Injections of oxytetracyclin 5 g IV for 3 days is reported to have given good results.

Diagnosis

Smears of milk may show chains of streptococci or staphylococci in smears of milk stained with methylene blue (1%) or Gram staining (Fig. 15.1a).

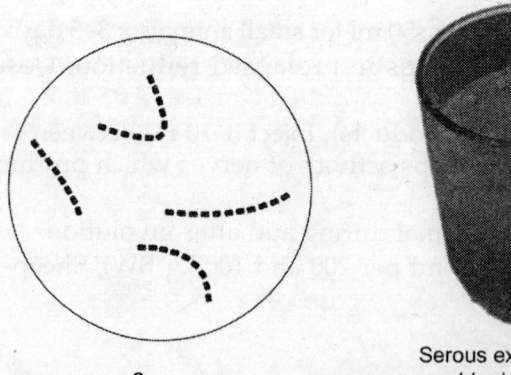
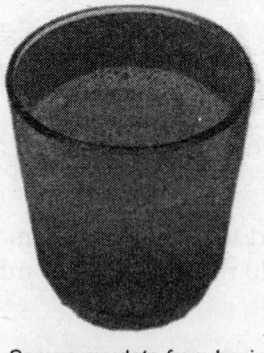
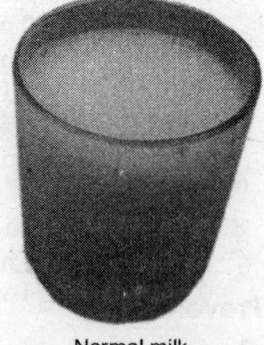

a

Serous exudate from bovine udder in filiform mastitis

Normal milk

b

Figs 15.1a and b: Gram staining

Masti Test (Mastitis field test kit of HiMedia)

This is a lab free test kit (field test)

Vaccines against mastitis are not successful. Excellent vigilance and rapid culling is the best method.

Treatment

1. For mycoplasmal mastitis which occurs as an outbreak, erythromycin, tylosin, tetracycline, quindine, and chloramphenicol work better, particularly tylosin which can be given in water or brown sugar.
2. There is a wide range of antibiotics for treatment and control of mastitis.
3. *Akyciceph Forte (Brihans)* is reported to be good to treat *E. coli* mastitis. It is injected 10 ml on alternate days. It is amikacin sulphate. If udder is inflamed and hard, inject isoflud 5 ml on first day.
   Dose of Akayci is 8–10 ml in cows given by IM route on alternate days (5, 10, 30, and 100 ml vials).
4. *Bovizox* (Ceftizoxime of Zydus).
5. 'Enrodac 10' injection of Hester. This contains enrofloxacin with wide range of action, including mycoplasma and other bacteria. Dose is 5 mg per kg BW or 1 ml/20 kg BW in all animals, by IM or IV route. May be extended for 7 to 10 days.
6. *Lykacetin injection (Lyka)* 3 g vial. Dose: 2–4 mg/kg BW IV or 20–30 mg/kg BW IM for 3–4 days.
7. *M. Ceft injection (Alembic):* 5 mg/kg BW to be given by IV route; contains ceftizoxime sodium. Single shot mastitis treatment.
8. *Floxidin vet (MSD/Intervet)*: Floxidin 10%, daily IM injection 2.5–5 mg/kg BW, IM for 3–4 days.

Anti-inflammatory treatment

1. Vetoprofen (Ketoprofen) IM, IV injection; 2–4 mg/kg BW till inflammation and swelling subside (3–5 days).
2. IT IS-M ointment (Van Vet product) for mastitis; 25 g tube, apply daily after milking.
3. Pyridase oral bolus (Cargil product), nimesulide and paracetamol. Cows—2 boli twice daily.
4. *Infla Gel (Neospark):* Herbal anti-inflammatory gel; 50 ml and 100 ml gel. Prophylactic and supportive for mastitis treatment.
5. *Megludyne (Flunixinmeglumine injection):* 1–2 ml injection per 25 kg BW by slow IV or IM injection.
6. Mastilep—a herbal gel. Should be used for massage on udder before parenteral therapy.
7. Wisprec spray is similar to Mastilep.

Preventive

1. *Amunty*: Nutritional immunity booster (Virbac Animal health). Contains vitamins, chelated minerals and antioxidants. Give 1 sachet daily in last month of pregnancy. It prevents mastitis.
2. *Uniselit (Ayurvet Ltd):* 10 g sachet to be given as Amunty.

Comprehensive Udder Healthcare Solutions for Prevention, Detection, Control, and Treatment of Mastitis

1. Special supplement for high demand period.

Uniselit: premix. It is a scientific combination of antioxidants and trace minerals containing vitamin E, selenium, zinc, manganese, copper, cobalt, calcium, phosphorus, and crude proteins.

Indications

a. Peak lactation requirements
b. Cotherapy of mastitis
c. Increased requirement for pregnancy
d. Enhances udder immunity by antioxidant action
e. Checks recurrence of mastitis, checks ROP.

Presentation: 10 g sachets

Dose: Cow, buffalo, horse: 1 sachet

Sheep, goat, pig: half sachet

To be given orally, once daily for 15 days.

2. *Mastilep gel:* Mastilep is a herbal gel (Ayurvet) which controls subclinical mastitis, supports clinical mastitis therapy, and is preventive for postparturient udder oedema.

Method of use: Wash the udder and teats thoroughly with water after each milking. Cover the udder and teats with gel twice daily for 5 days postcalving.

Package: 125 g lamitube in monocarton.

3. *Mastrip:* It is a quick solution to detect subclinical, clinical and advanced subclinical mastitis so that preventive medication may be started. It is a booklet containing strips of indicator paper which is to be dipped in milk. The colour which develops can be matched with the coloured comparator strip which shows all the above conditions. (Ayurvet product)

Blue = clinical mastitis

Green = advanced subclinical mastitis

Light or parrot green = subclinical mastitis

Golden yellow = normal udder

4. *Mastidip (Ayurvet product):* It is a post-milking teat disinfectant of teats.

Use: Mix Mastidip fluid and water in ratio of 1 : 2 to make about 150 ml of mixture. After washing the teats, dip teats for a short-time in the solution.

Packing: 100 ml bottle.

Infusions

1. *Pendistrin-SH (Zydus):* Contains procain penicillin, streptomycin sulphate sulfamerazine. Introduce contents of one tube every 12 hours or after each milking for 3 milkings in acute and chronic mastitis.

2. *Uddercef (Zydus):* 3.5 g prefilled syringe contains cefuroxime sodium 250 ml. For clinical and subclinical mastitis. Infuse the drug into the affected quarter after milking (3 successive milkings) by the syringe filled with medicine.

Sprays and Teat Dips

Mastilep (Herbal gel and spray, Ayurvet Ltd): 125 ml spray; 50 and 125 g gel tubes.

Mastidip (Ayurvet—100 ml liquid): For moisturising and disinfecting teats and milkers' hands for preventing mastitis.

Wisprec (Natural Remedies): It is a herbal spray for udder to control inflammation in mastitis.

Ceftiofur and Enroflexacin are drugs of choice for *E. coli* mastitis.

Homoeopathy

Homoeopathy is cheap and effective for treatment of acute and chronic mastitis.

1. *In early acute stage:* When the udder becomes red and swollen, Bryonia 200 works well. It may be given at the rate of 1 teaspoonful morning and evening.
2. If blood is mixed with milk then give Phosphorus 200 after an hour or more.
3. In chronic fibrotic mastitis with milk looking like whitish pus, give Hepar Sulph 200, 1 teaspoonful in morning and 1 tsp in daytime and 1 tsp in evening.
   Also, give Silicia 200 3 times, and the same frequency works for Hepar Sulph but keep a margin of 20–30 minutes between the two medicines.
4. Phytolacca 1000 may be given once in a week (1 tsp) if the udder becomes very hard.
5. In cases where milk yield stops due to thick puslike exudates, then giving 1 tsp of Silicia 200 and 1 tsp of Hepar Sulph liquids at 15 minutes gap to start the puslike material to flow out on milking on the next day.

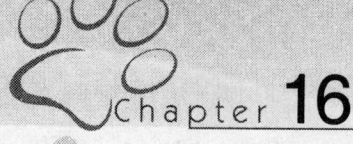

Chapter 16

Udder Diseases other than Mastitis

■ BLOOD IN MILK

Blood in milk may come due to any kind of visible or invisible injury to udder which is highly vascular. Blood may disappear in 2–3 days but if it persists, take body temperature. If it is normal, give the following medicines:

1. *Adchrome injection*, 30 ml vial (G. Loucatos, Co): Inject 5 ml, IM daily till blood in milk stops.
2. *Novizac injection (Vanvet Co):* This is reported to stop bleeding from anywhere in the body including blood in milk. Novizac is mixed with 20 ml ATP stimulator which makes 50 ml. Inject 25 ml by IV, IM, or SC route for 2 days.
3. *Styplon bolus (Himalaya):* It is a bolus which can stop bleeding of any kind besides blood with milk such as epistaxis (bleeding from nose), uterine bleeding, bleeding from stomach (haemoptysis), etc. or postoperative bleeding.
   Cow, buffalo, horse, camel—1–2 boli morning and evening
   Calves and foals—1 bolus twice a day
   Sheep and goats—1/2 bolus twice a day
   Packing: 1 strip of 4 bolus.
4. *Homoeopathic:* Phosphorus 200: by mouth
   1 teaspoonful 3 times a day in cow, buffalo. 8–10 drops in dogs for vomiting of blood or bloody diarrhea (wonderful even in terminal stage). Repeat at 20 minutes, 30 minutes.
5. *Ethamsylate injection (Tineta):* 5–10 mg per kg BW as SC/IM injection.
   Injected at dose rate of 15–20 ml for large animals and 1–3 ml in small animals by SC or IM route. Will also stop bleeding in milk.
6. *Bloodren capsules (Epicon Labs):* Large animal 10 capsules twice a day; small animal 5 capsules.

■ OEDEMA OF UDDER

Oedema of udder is physiological at parturition but it may get aggravated particularly in periparturient heifers. It is more common if grain feeding is not reduced during last few weeks of pregnancy. Oedema may become too severe and extend to thighs, perineum and external genitalia or even brisket area.

Treatment

1. *Serokind Plus (Mankind):* It contains seraptopeptidase paracetamol and meloxicam.
   Dose: 2 bolus daily for 2–5 days in large animals; 1 bolus daily for 2–5 days in small animals.
2. *Romat:* Inject 10 ml/day by IM route once daily for 3 days.

3. *Avil:* Inject 10 ml once a day for 3 days.
4. *Redema:* Inject 10 ml once a day for 3 days.
5. *Isoflud:* 5–10 ml, IM daily for 2–3 days.

METRITIS

Inflammation of uterus. Metritis is a common disease following ROP, prolapse, AI or parturition or abortion. Any of the common pyogenic organisms or gram-negative anaerobes may cause it. Other uncommon causes are *Actinobacterium pyogenes, Fusobacterium necrophorum* and Prevotella species. (See also chapter on pyometra and ROP).

Symptoms

Pyometritis, purulent discharge with sometimes infertility.

Treatment

In uterine pus, minimum inhibitory concentration is difficult to attain therefore cephalosporins are preferred over oxytetracyclin. *Hyterus* (Kepler Vety Mission Pvt Ltd, Ahmedabad); Bolus contain Nitrofurazone 60 mg, Metronidazole 100 mg, povidone iodine, 60 mg; urea 6 gm. Insert by hand 2 or 4 boluses into each horn and repeat after 24 hours.

Ural (Alembic): It is a liquid available in syringe, effective in presence of pus. 10 g prefilled syringe with a long applicator (tube) is used to push liquid via cervix. It is used once or twice daily for 3–5 days.

Xceft (Alembic): 250 mg vial contains ceftiofur sodium with 5 ml distilled water for injection. It is good for canine pyometra (Open cervix or closed cervix). Dosage is 1.1 to 2.2 mg per kg BW for 3 to 5 days.

Ceft Plus (Lyka) injection: 3 g and 4.5 g vials of ceftriaxone sodium.

Dose: 5–10 mg/kg BW once or twice a day by IM, IV, or SC route for 3–5 days.

Lyphos Vet (Lyka): Phosphorus injection (Toldim Phos).

Dose: Large animals: 5–15 ml.
Small animals: 1–3 ml.

Inflavet Plus (Virbac): To minimize inflammation.

Dose: Large animals: 1 tab morning and evening.

Small animals: 1/4 to 1/2 tab morning and evening.

Homoeopathic

1. Hepar Sulph 200—1 teaspoonful three times a day on alternate days for cow (orally).
2. Silicia 200—1 teaspoonful three times a day orally.
   Dogs—10 drops twice a day is enough.
   Silicia 200 can be given with Hepar Sulph 200 with a gap of 20 minutes also 3 times a day orally to expel pus in cows. In dogs, 10 drops 3 times a day may be given orally.

■ MILK FEVER (PARTURIENT PARESIS) (Hypocalcaemia, Calving Paralysis)

This is a metabolic disease. Although the name has 'fever' added to it, in fact there is no milk and no fever.

The main cause is deficiency of calcium due to lot of it secreted out in milk and enough going to bones of foetus. Normally, the cows and buffaloes have 10 mg% calcium which drops in this condition to 2 to 7 mg%. The problem may occur at any age but usually, it occurs 10 days after calving or it may occur 2–3 months after calving, particularly in high milk yielders. It can also occur due to inadequate food or neglect during transport. The disease is more common in winter and spring.

Factors

1. Colostrum contains 12 to 13 times more calcium than in the blood.
2. Inadequate calcium in feed even before calving.
3. Blood Ca: Magnesium ratio normally is 6:1. If Ca goes down and magnesium goes up, the cow is down and looks unconscious. If calcium goes down and magnesium is normal then the cow mostly remains on ground and can stand with great difficulty. If Ca and Mg both go down then convulsions or twitching of muscles start even in lying position.

Three Stages

Prepartum Stage

1. Muscle spasm in legs and neck, excitement.
2. Loss of appetite.
3. Tossing about the head.
4. Tongue hangs out of mouth.
5. Temperature normal or slightly elevated.

Second stage/Sternal recumbancy

1. The neck is turned back towards abdomen.
2. Muzzle becomes dry.
3. Cow cannot stand.
4. Eyes become dry and the pupils become dilated.
5. Heartbeat goes up to 75 or 80 per minute. Pulse becomes weak and heart sounds feeble.
6. Constipation and poor ruminal motility.

Third Stage

In this stage there is paralysis-like effect. Temperature is subnormal, heartbeat and blood circulation start failing. Heartbeat may be 120/minute but the heart sounds are feeble and weak. The animal is laterally recumbent and unable to sit up. Feeble circulation results in oliguria or anuria (effect on kidney circulation). Pulse becomes weak. Recombancy may lead to bloat or tympany.

Hypocalcaemia with *hypomagnesemia* may result in muscular convulsions and tetanic spasms and twitching of eyelids. If there is hypophosphatemia as well then calcium therapy may give response but not enough to make the cow stand.

Clinical Findings

1. Calcium below 9–11 mg/dl.
2. In mild cases magnesium in blood may be normal but low or high in severe case.
3. Serum phosphorus goes down to as low as 1.5–3 mg/dl.
4. Blood glucose may remain normal but if ketosis also develops, it may also go down.
5. WBCs: Eosionpenia (may be up to 0%)
   Lymphopenia
   Neutrophilia (due to relative lymphopenia)
   These changes are observed in late stage due to stress resulting in corticosteroid secretion which destroys eosinophils and lymphocytes.

Guiding Symptoms (Diagnosis)

1. Paresis (partial paralysis and narcosis, or semiconscious condition)—hypocalcaemia and hypermagnesemia.
2. Paddling of hind legs in recumbent (downer) cow and recumbancy—with or without paresis = hypocalcaemia + normal magnesium.
3. Paddling and tetany of hind and forelimbs + hyperesthesia (sensitive to touch and sound) the cow may later beome recumbent = hypocalcaemia + hypomagnesemia.

   Some cows respond to calcium therapy; if not, give phosphorus to give energy to muscle (high energy phosphate bonds) in the form of Tonophosphan or Urimin or Catasole injections.

   The cause of milk fever is not well-understood hence judicious line of treatment should be followed. Although calcium shortage is at the center or key point of disease because 12 times normal calcium comes out in the colostrum. Therefore, 12 times the normal calcium must be replaced.

Treatment

1. *"Speed Up"(Natural Remedies):* Bottle, oral 800 g: After calcium Boro gluconate injection IV, feed/drench 535 g (2/3rd) bottle of speed up to the affected cow/buffalo. Remaining 1/3rd (265 g) may be fed as 2nd dose 10–12 hours after the first dose.
   Speed up contains ionic calcium hence is very quickly absorbed in 15 minutes and maintains Ca blood level for longer period. It also protects the heart against high blood calcium. Thirdly, it provides instant energy. Absorption starts in rumen (nonionic Ca needs 12 to 16 hours for absorption).
2. *Inomilk (Hester product):* Ca and phosphorus product. Facilitates easy let down of milk.
   Dose: Cows, etc.—50 ml twice a day
3. *Intacal-IM (Bovicura/Intas product):* It contains calcium, D_3, and B_{12}. It can prevent chances of milk fever and supportive after IV calcium in milk fever. (Presentation 45 ml vial)
   Dose: 10–15 ml 3 times a week for 2 weeks before parturition.
4. *Ultracal (30 ml injection):* Use as for Intacal IM.
5. *Milk Fever Formula (Zydus):* 450 ml injection. Use as instructed by the manufacturer.

6. *Vibra Cal Gel (Neospark product):* It prevents hypocalcaemia, milk fever, improves milk production, normal calving and expulsion of placenta. It can be given along with IV calcium injection. Vibra Cal Gel is available as gel of 250 ml. It contains calcium, phosphorus, cobalt, thiamine, niacin, pantothenic acid, vitamins A, D, E, C, riboflavin, B$_{12}$, selenium, and energy.

   Dose: Give one tube at first sign of calving, second tube at 6–12 hours post-calving. Repeat at 12 hours, if needed.

   For regular milk yield: Give 50–70 ml/cow/day for 5–10 days.

7. *Balanion powder (Zydus):* 50 g daily for 10 days before parturition and 10 days after parturition.

   Cobacal-D (Cargil product): Ionic Ca, D$_3$, and B$_{12}$.

   Prepartum—10–15 ml IM thrice a week.

   Postpartum—same as above, IM for 2 weeks.

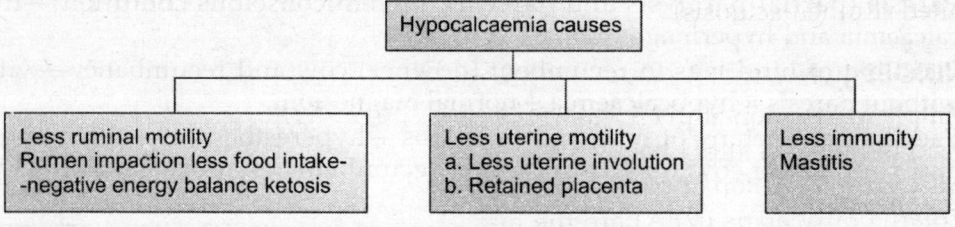

Other drugs/injections are listed in Index of drugs.

Chapter 17

Diseases of Rumen

In adult ruminants the stomach occupies about 75% of the abdominal cavity and the biggest of the four compartments is Rumen. Rumen has fluid pH of 6.5 to 7, ideal for the normal, crores of helpful bacteria and protozoa. Any abnormal shift in pH will make the ruminant sick. Example at pH 5.5 or less the protozoa get completely inhibited (Rumen acidosis).

■ INDIGESTION

- Simple indigestion at pH 5.5 to 7.5.
- Acid indigestion at pH below 5.5.
- Alkaline indigestion at pH 7.5 to 8.5.

Volatile fatty acids (VFA) are the main acids which regulate the pH of rumen besides lactic, butygric acid, etc.

Simple Indigestion

This is due to altered pH, generally about 5.5 to 7.5 due to production of much lactic acid. Main symptoms are loss of muzzle moisture, stopped rumination, and poor appetite but rule out fever.

Treatment

If pH is acidic then it has to be neutralised with buffers such as:

1. *Buffzone (Intas):* Contains buffers and metabolic boosters.
   Dose: Cows and buffaloes 200 g.
   Calves and heifers: 60–80 g; sheep, goats 50 g daily for 3–4 days.
2. *Rumbuf (Rumen buffer with live yeast; Merial product):* It removes ruminal acidosis, maintains normal pH, supports useful microflora (packing of 200 g).
   Dose: Cow, buffalo 200 g for 3–4 days.
   Calves/heifers 100 g for 3–4 days.
   Sheep, goats 50 g for 3–4 days.
3. *Actisaf powder (Merial product):* Live heat stable (pallets) yeast (1×10^{10} CFU/g)
   Action: Acidosis control, improves milk yield, indigestion and results in weight gain in calves.
   Dose: Cows/buffalows 5 g; calf 2 g; sheep, goat 3 g orally for 2–3 days (packing of 150 g, 500 g, 5 and 25 kg).
4. *Biobloom:* Highest bypass protein and enzymes, Saccharomyces, Lactobacillus, and protein more than 50%.

Biobloom reduces lactic acidosis, helps in digestion and promotes rumen microflora and inhibits harmful bacteria. Highly palatable, improves all-round rumen health.

Dose: Calf 5 g/day; cows 15 g/day (packing of 250 g and 1 kg).

5. *Rumistim (Neospark):* This contains about 15 herbs (as a 45 g food cake). It is useful for simple indigestion ruminal stasis (impaction) and anorexia (loss of appetite).
   Dose: Cows, buffaloes, camels—one feed cake orally for 2–4 days. Sheep and goats 1/2 cake for 2–4 days.

6. *Floratone bolus* (Concept product): It contains sodium bi. carb., mag. trisilicate methionine, yeast, nicotine, cobalt, copper, ginger, gention, and sod. phosph.
   Indications: Simple indigestion, poor microflora (impaction) and rumen atony (impaction) means stoppage of rumination.
   Dose: Adult bovines 1 bolus 3 times or 12 hourly.

7. *Perinorm injection (Ipca):* Comes in packing of 2 ml and 10 ml; tablets 1 × 10.
   This can prove very good complimentary drug. It induces ruminal or intestinal movement if there is ruminal stasis (lump formation in rumen). 2 ml injection may be given IM or IV, twice a day. This may start rumination and is very good.

8. *Rumeric injection (Virbac, 10 and 20 ml vials):* Contains lipotropic amino acids and nicotinamide. This is supportive treatment for indigestion and liver dysfunction.
   Dose: Cattle, sheep, and goats 1 ml per 40 kg BW by IM/IV route for 3–5 days.

9. *Provisac Plus (Provimi product):* It helps management of ruminal acidosis and indigestion. It contains probiotic enzymes and minerals.
   Dose: 2–4 boli daily, orally.

Follow-up Treatment

1. Give attention to feed and water. Feed should be balanced and *free from fungal toxins* which are mostly produced in cakes having more than 10% moisture.
2. Stop too much feeding of *poor quality dry grass* having indigestible fiber.
3. Test the drinking water because *too much of hard water* kills normal rumen microflora. 'Aquadur sensitive' which are test strips manufactured by Macherey-Nagel (Germany) are available from Fisher Scientific, Product code M0210, 403-404 B wing, Delphi Hiranandani Park, Powai, Mumbai 400076. Tel: 18002097001. (₹ 3174 for about 100 sticks). This can determine water hardness of 5, 10, and 20 ppm with a single strip.
4. *Rumen FS powder (Alembic):* It is for antiacidosis, antilaminitis, and digestion support (100 g sachet).
   Dose: 100 g/day/animal.
5. *Rumisacc bolus (Zydus) 4 boli × 30 strips box:* 4 enzymes, liver extract, ginger, 6 amino acids, 4 probiotics + rumen buffer, and soya bean meal compose it.
   Dose: 2–4 boli for 3 to 5 days.
   Indication: Anorexia, mild bloat, impaction of rumen.

▓ ACID INDIGESTION

Acid indigestion is mainly due to the following causes:

1. Accidental or ignorant act of feeding of excess of carbohydrate food (rice, wheat, maize, jwar, potatoes, etc.) suddenly.

2. Decomposed food or silage, bread, apples, etc.
3. Hotel waste food.
4. Sudden change of food, mainly carbohydrates or vegetable food such as sorghum and wheat, etc.
   (Synonyms—Lactic acidemia, sudden death syndrome, rumen acidosis, wheat poisoning).

Findings

1. Ruminal fluid pH goes down to 5 or less.
2. High osmolarity of ruminal fluid from 6.9 to 20 or 25.
3. Marked dehydration due to fluid oozing from blood into rumen.
4. Haemoconcentration due to loss of fluid from blood.
5. Atony of rumen by acidic pH.
6. Release of histamine.
7. Release of toxic things *like methane and endotoxins*.
8. *Fall in urine pH* (acidic) due to acidosis (normally alkaline).
9. *Cerebrocortical necrosis due to thiaminase enzyme.* pH of fluid can be detected by pH papers of any manufacturer.

Symptoms

1. Dull, anorexia 8–12 hours after faulty food.
2. Dull, depressed.
3. Rumen with fluid.
4. Kicking of abdomen due to pain.
5. Grunting sound and grinding of teeth due to pain.
6. Pulse rate of 100–120/minute (very high).
7. Acidic urine or even anuria (no urination).
8. There may be 'milk fever' like turning of head towards abdomen.
9. Eyes sunken due to dehydration.
10. Faecal pH 4.4 to 7.0 (low).

Treatment

1. *Give saline purgatives* like *magnesium sulphate.*
2. *Give alkalisers* such as sodium bicarbonate (floratone bolus given under simple indigestion)or inject 2.5 to 5% sodium bicarbonate (500 ml or 1000 ml by IV route slowly in adult cow and less in calf.
3. *Give antihistaminics* (Anistamine injection of Intas or 'Avil' injection (30 ml vial of Hoechst or Avilin Vet, MSD).
4. *Inject thiamine hydrochloride.* 'B com vet' injection of Lyka which contains 100 mg of thiamine (10 ml injection/day besides other B vitamins. Give 10 injections.)
5. *'Beejet'100 ml injection* (Vets Pharma) or Plexovet of Eldin Pharma 33.3 mg thiamin plus other B vitamins (Dose: large animals 10–15 ml; small animals 9–10 ml.

ALKALINE INDIGESTION

Alkaline indigestion is relatively less common. Generally, it is due to high protein food which produces alkaline ammonia (gas) which forms ammonium hydroxide with water.

Causes

1. Urea—as a part of feed.
2. High protein food.
3. Consumption of plants rich in protein (soya bean, berseem, etc.).
4. Eating of placenta postcalving.
5. Sudden change to protein-rich diet (oilseed cakes, soya bean, etc.).
6. Eating of decomposed oil cakes.
7. Excessive paddy straw for long-time.

Symptoms

1. *Anorexia (off feed)*
2. Suspended rumination and continuous *drooling of saliva*
3. *Muscular tremors or convulsions due to ammonia in blood* (toxic to brain) which is beyond the capacity of liver to detoxify.

Diagnosis

1. High blood urea nitrogen 15 to 70 mg%
2. High ruminal fluid pH (above 7.5%)
3. Ammonical odour in ruminal fluid

Treatment

If early treatment is started within 2–3 days then complete recovery is possible.

1. *Correct ruminal pH:* Give 5–10% acetic acid at the rate of 5–10 ml per kg BW. Roughly 250 to 500 ml solution orally or intraruminally. I have found this quite good, particularly in cattle who have ingested plastic from city roads.
2. Administer oral antibiotics to stop multiplication of harmful, ammonia or toxin producing bacteria growing in alkaline (abnormal) pH. I used to give Ciflox TZ (Intas) tablets in jaggary @ 1 tablet per 50 kg BW (half of normal dose) for 2 days.
   Or
3. Steclin (tetracyclin bolus, Zydus product) 500 mg bolus @ 1 bolus/day for 2 days
4. Lykadin bolus (sulphadimidine of Lyka) Give 1 bolus per 50 kg BW for 2 days
5. *Rumi Stim (45 g feed cake of Neospark):* It contains herbal compounds which start ruminal movement and start digestion.
   Give 1 feed cake per cow/buffalo and 1/2 to calf, sheep and goats. Or Lact Yeast gel of the same company may be fed at the same rate.
6. *Feed Well gel (Neospark):* Nutritional and vitamins, lactobacillus and saccharomyces cerviciae. Give 1 tube orally per animal for 1 to 2 days. Or give Ecotas boli @ 2 boli/animal/day × 4 days.
7. Perinorm injection (see under acid indigestion) or Perinorm tablet (1 or 2) per day till recovery.
8. Give Mifex or Intalyte IV to stimulate ruminal movement and for energy.

■ SUBACUTE RUMINAL ACIDOSIS (SARA)

SARA is less common but may occur due to slow exposure to the same factors which animals are exposed to such as slow feeding of grains, surplus wheat, or much feeding of leguminous plants (soya bean, pulses, peanuts, etc.).

Line of treatment is the same as for ruminal acidosis with slight variation. In such cases, preventive measures whould be taken.

1. *Rumi Buff* (Neospark product): Rumi Buff contains buffers, alkalisers, linseed, ginger, gention (appetizer), fenugreek (methi), and capsicum. This drug normalises ruminal environment and function. One of the best drugs.
2. *Perinorm (Ipca)*: Give Perinorm 10 mg tablets (1 per calf, 2 per adult) once or twice a day till return to normal. Or give 2 ml Perinorm injection morning and evening.
3. Correct the feed given.
4. In dairy farms it may be due to toxins in feed. In such cases, it is advised to give mycotoxin binder and see the results.
   Example: Immutox (Intas): It contains HSCAS toxin binder (25 kg bag). Add 1.5 kg per tonne feed.
   Mytox nil (Lyka product in packing of 1 kg): This removes moisture and pathogens and helps digestion
   Dose: Large animal 30 g/day.
      Small animal 15 g/day.
5. *Rumen FS powder*: Instant buffer (Alembic product, 100 g sachet)
   Dose: 100 g/animal/day. Contains buffers, minerals, vitamins, probiotic, and live yeast.
6. *Bioboost powder (Lyka)*: It keeps rumen pH between 6.2 and 6.7 and helps in digestion of fibres and enhances milk yield.
   Dose: Cow 10 g per day
      Small animals 5 g per day
7. *Provisacc Plus*: For mild rumen acidosis. It is a combination of yeast Saccharomyces and lactobacillus, methionine, zinc, copper, cobalt.
   Use: Mild rumen acidosis, indigestion, chronic anorexia.
   Dose: 2 boli twice daily for 3–5 days.

■ IMPACTION OF RUMEN

Accumulation of food material of dry, moistureless and without gas is called impaction. Hosts are cattle, buffaloes, sheep and goats.

Causes

Feeding of exceedingly dry and unnutritious grass, plants or straw and dry grain mixture. The impacted food gets deprived of protozoa and bacterial population which carry on normal digestion. Impacted food putrefies and liberates toxins. There is atony of rumen and atrophy of ruminal wall (muscles). This atony is reversible for 2–3 days only. Eating plastic sheets or bags from street or garbage also causes impaction.

Signs

There is gradual distension of abdomen, loss of appetite. Rumen part (left) of abdomen in hard and doughy (pits on pressure). Usually faeces are not passed out or are scanty, hard balls are passed out. Death may occur due to negative energy balance (subnormal body temperature) and dehydration.

Treatment

1. Drench 500 to 1000 ml of linseed oil by stomach tube. If not possible, give mustard oil, about 500 ml.
2. Inject Perinorm 2–3 ml IV in morning and after 6–8 hours.
3. Administer rumenotoric (we use Rumentas of Intas) which contains Antimony pot. Tartrate, a motility inducer, ferrous sulphate, copper sulphate, and cobalt chloride.
   Dose: Large animals 2 boli daily.
   Small animals 1 bolus, daily, orally.
4. Administer Biobloom bolus (Zydus) which contains Saccharomyces cerveciae, lactobacillus, protein, phytase, cellulose, xylanase, pectinase, calcium, phosphorus, protein, carbohydrates, vitamins, etc. It stimulates useful ruminal bacterial growth and is also highly palatable.
   Or give Rumibuff or Bovilax (Neospark or Pachoplus bolus of Dabur—use these as Biobloom.
5. Administer intravenously the following mixture:
   i. Tribivet M injection (Intas) or Hitone injection (Lyka) 5 ml.
   ii. Tonophosphan injection 15–20 ml IV once daily.
6. *Next day or by evening:* Protein C liquid (Hester product) at the following dose rate: 100 ml daily for 10 days.
7. *Preventive:* Tonoricin (30 ml injection of Vetoquinol Co)
   Dose: For acute case 10–25 ml SC, IM or IV injection
   Or Metabolin (SC, IM or IV injection), a Hester product, in the same dose as for Tonoricin.
   Presentation of 30 ml and 100 ml
8. *Ruchi Boost (Vanvet):* A pasty, palatable, honey based appetizer. It may be applied on lips for licking.
9. *Impacdon (Vets Pharma):* It is a herbal product. It alone is said to be 'superb'.
   Dose: Cow/buffalo: 100–200 g BD; calf, etc. 50–100 g BD; sheep/goat 25–50 g BD.

▓ RUMINAL TYMPANY (BLOAT) PRIMARY

The primary kind can be of two types, frothy and gaseous.

Causes (Brief)

1. Too much green plants or grass feeding or feeding of fermentable carbohydrates like cabbage, potatoes, beans, bananas, etc.
2. Lack of roughages.
3. High calcium and low phosphorus in diet.
4. Plant toxins, HCN, leguminous plants or plants which retard belching (Pasture bloat).
5. Toxic gases in rumen; methane, CO_2, carbon monoxide, etc.
6. Secondary bloat is due to obstruction by foreign bodies, stenosis, etc.

Signs

Respiratory rate becomes high as also pulse or heart rate; grinding of teeth, loss of appetite; bloated abdomen; protrusion of tongue. Mortality is generally around 1%.

Treatment

Withdraw all foods and water
1. If in a village, give the following to expel gases:
   a. Turpentine oil 15–20 ml.
   b. Linseed or mustard oil, 500 ml.
   c. Asaefoetida (Heeng), about 0.5 to 1 g. Administer by stomach tube or by careful drenching.
2. Formalin—Give 10 to 30 ml diluted with about 250–300 ml water, orally.

Allopathic Medicines

1. Rumicare vet powder 125 g sachet, twice daily.
2. *Tympax:* 100 ml suspension; Vets Pharma.
3. *Tympfree suspension (Zydus):* Contains Simethicone in oil base.
   Dose: Cattle/buffalo—100 ml orally; repeat after 6 hours if needed.
   Sheep and goats—50 ml.
   Give by stomack tube or by 100 ml bottle.
4. *Vayuhara (Novartis):* Same as for Tympfree.
5. *Afnil (Dabur):* Herbal. Also acts on frothy bloat.
   Dose: 50 ml twice daily for 2 days.
6. *Bloatosil:* Contains dimethicone; dose 100 ml/cow.
7. *Gasbl (Kepler):* Contains Simethicone.
   Dose: 100 ml twice a day in cows.
8. *Bloatarid (Intas product; 100 ml bottle):* Simethicone + MgOH + sorbitol + aluminium hydroxid.
   Dose: Orally 100 ml for cattle.
   20 ml for sheep and goats.
9. *Tyrel (Natural Remedies):* Liquid herbal medicine.
   Dose: 40 ml twice a day.
   Herbal drugs act slowly hence simethicone containing drugs may be used first, then others.

■ GRUNTING IN CATTLE

Grunting or painful sound with or without grinding of teeth is seen in case of the following diseases:
1. *Diseases of chest:*
   a. Severe pneumonia
   b. Pleurisy
   c. Pulmonary emphysema.
2. *Diseases of abdomen:*
   a. Bloat
   b. Intestinal obstruction
   c. Abomasitis

    d. Peritonitis

    e. Enterotoxemia (sheep and goat)

    f. Plastic impaction in rumen.

■ LEFT-SIDED DISPLACEMENT OF ABOMASUM (LDA)

LDA is due to several factors but the main factor is feeding highly concentrated diet 2 weeks before parturition or 2 to 4 weeks after parturition. Lack of roughages hypocalcaemia and ketosis are also causal factors. Up to 20% cows with LDA and diarrhoea may die.

Signs

Loss of appetite, ketosis, generally in 4 to 7 years old cows. It is more common in spring season. Hypocalcaemia is usually seen. Gas accumulates in the abomasums, methane makes 70% of the gas and the rest is carbon dioxide. Milk production drops. Fatty degeneration of liver is quite common.

Tests

1. *Ketone in urine may* be positive.
2. *AST values* between 100 and 180 U/L.
3. *Betahydroxybutyrate* 1000 to 1600 μmol/L.
4. *High PCV and high haemoglobin* are present due to haemoconcentration.

Prevention

1. Maximise dry matter intake in terminal stages of pregnancy.
2. Avoid negative energy balance (hypothermia).

Treatment

1. Injections of perinorm.
2. Injections of CBG (calcium borogluconate).
3. Surgical—replacing abomasums surgically.
4. Supportive—Ionic calcium orally such as speed up 500 ml (Natural Remedies) or Hyporid powder 90 g/day. Hypocalcaemia promotes LDA.

Feed Ingredients to be Aware of

1. *Oxallate rich*: Too much oxalates bind calcium in the AGI tract to form insoluble calcium oxalate causing wastage or loss of calcium, e.g. Paddy straw, Pusa giant.
2. *Phytic acid*: Phytic acid binds with several minerals, such as iron, zinc, calcium, phosphorus to form insoluble complexes and excretion in faeces.
   For examples, leguminous hays, oil seeds, and cereals. To neutralize their effect, phytase is included in some feed supplements which destroys phytic acid.
3. *Toxic minerals: Arsenic*: source is insecticidal dips, sprays, etc. Result is acute gastroenteritis, diarrhoea, and nervous incoordination.

■ TOXICOSIS

Selenium: Soils may be rich in selenium so also the forage plants but these plants are wild and unpalatable. Symptoms are dyspnoea, diarrhoea, and death. In chronic form, the disease is called 'Blind staggers' or 'Alkali disease'. Presence of 10 mg per kg of feed is considered toxic.

Symptoms

Loss of hairs from switch of the tail or even tip of the tail may be lost.

▓ FLUORINE TOXICITY

This may occur through fluorine-rich water or feed.

Symptoms

Browning of teeth, pitting and attrition of teeth, arthritis, and deformed bone. Slaked lime treatment with 500–1000 mg per liter water is then allowed to settle for 6 days. This can reduce 90% of fluorine from water.

▓ MOLYBDENUM

Grasses having 3–10 mg per kg of feed are toxic. Symptoms are due to binding and loss of copper. Main symptoms are of copper deficiency such as anaemia, loss of colour of hair and chronic diarrhoea.

▓ COPPER

Source of poison is copper rich soils, copper containing chemicals ($CuSO_4$) or in mineral mixtures. Main sign is haemoglobinuria and anaemia. Toxic level is 3.5 mg/kg BW or above. Sheep are most susceptible.

Treatment

Give 100 mg of ammonium molybdate or 1 g of anhydrous sodium sulfate to lambs to excrete the excess copper.

▓ BYPASS FEED INGREDIENTS

Some of the doctors may not be aware of the extreme usefulness of nutrients by 'bypass' technology.

In the rumen, many of the major feed ingredients undergo too much loss or wastage by rumen microflora and as much as 60–80% protein, fat, carbohydrates may be lost in rumen by rumen microflora hence nowadays these substances are coated with substances which protect these molecules to about 70–80% extent and which are digested in abomasum and utilised to be available for animal growth and production at low cost.

Examples of bypass feeds available in India:
1. *Cafplan (Bovicura/Intas):* Bypass, fat, protein, starch, chromium and yeast
   Dose: 100 g/day cow, etc. (pack of 3 kg).
2. *HFM (Hester)*
   Dose: 100 g daily or 1 to 1.5% feed to increase milk fat percentage (presentation of 1, 5, and 20 kg).
3. Khurak (bypass protein, fat with minerals, vitamins, and probiotics).
   I have found it to be very useful in poor health calves. It has very attractive falvour. It cures negative energy balance. One month before parturition it helps in normal delivery. It brings the animal to normal heat; increases milk yield.

      Dose: Lactating cows, etc. 150–300 g/animal/day
             Sheep/goats: 20–30 g/day/animal
             Pacxkings: 1.5 and 15 kg

4. *Nutri-Sacc (Cargil)*: Bypass protein, fat, energy, minerals, and vitamins (1 kg and 25 kg). Improves fat percent in milk.
   Dose: 5 gm per litre of milk yield (5 L—50 g).

5. *Hilak: Bypass fat,* (Ayurvet product): Improves fat percent in milk.
   Dose: 5 g per litre of milk yield (5 litres-50 g; 6–10 litres, 100 g; 11–15 litres, 150 g, above 15 litres, 200 g).
   To be given twice daily; orally, till desired results are obtained. Feeding in the last month of pregnancy gives good results.

6. *Galacshot: Bypass fat* + energy + herbal extracts; azadirecta, asparagus, and withania; 1 kg and 5 kg powder.
   *Dose:*10 g powder for more than 10 litres milk yield/day/animal or 100 g/day/animal, orally.

7. *M Power (Bovian)*: Contains bypass fat, protein, probiotics, vitamins, A, D_3, E, biotin, niacin, etc.
   Dose: Cows, etc.—100 g per day.

Fast Rumen Development

Quickrumi (Zydus, 200 g and 500 g): Product of coated sodium butyrate and lactic acid bacillus, to improve rumen development, quick weaning, improved digestion and absorption.

Dose: Age 10–30 days—15 g daily.
        31–60 days—20 g daily.
        61–90 days—25 g daily.
        Above 90 days—30 g/day.

Feed Components and Digestion

There are more than 2000 substances used for feeding cattle. They are subclassified into roughages and concentrates.
1. Concentrates: (a) Protein rich (b) Energy rich.
2. Roughages: (a) Dry (Straw, hay) (b) Green.

Greens

Cultivated green fodder contains about 2–3% digestible crude protein (DCP) and 10% total digestible nutrients (TDN). About 10 tonnes of greens can be obtained from on acre of land. Berseem and lucern are leguminous greens which contain about 3% DCP and 12% TDN and give higher yield of 300 quintals in multiple cuttings. These fodders are also poor in calcium and phosphorus and other minerals and proteins, hence supplemental feeding of concentrate mixtures is required for optimum yield.

    Jowar and Sudan grass and MP chari are good crops which yield up to 150 or 200 quintals of greens per acre. They are poor in proteins (0.5 to 1% DCP) but good in TDN (11 to 15%). Oat is very good fodder for dairy cows. It has 2 to 2.5% DCP and 17% TDN in wet basis.

Other good fodders are Napier grass, hybrid napier, paragrass and Guinea grass. These grasses grow well in summer and monsoon season and produce 30–40 tonnes per acre of land. Thus, 2 or 3 cows can be fed per acre of land.

Roughages

Hay and straws are two roughages which can be fed. Hay is carefully dried grass or fodder to reduce the moisture to 15 to 20% to inhibit spoilage by bacterial and fungal growth. Lucern or alfaalfa plants are best to make hay. Such hay contains 14 to 15% DCP and 50% TDN. Grasses, berseem and cowpea, etc. are not good to make hay which have thick stem, and are difficult to dry.

Straws

Straws are very poor in protein and minerals and rich in crude fibre. In developed countries, straws are not used for feeding but only as bedding material. Their DCP is negligible but TDN is about 40%. To make up for protein, minerals, etc. 1 to 2 kg of concentrate mixtures are added per animal per day. Mineral mixtures rich in calcium, phosphorus, copper, cobalt, zinc, and vitamins must be added to get good milk yield and disease resistance.

Leaves as fodder

Tree leaves contain good quantity of crude protein hence they can be fed in conditions of draught. Proven good leaves are Peepal (Fiscus religiosa), Babul (Acacia Arabica), Kachnar and Bel (Aegle marmelos).

Addition of 1.25% sodium hydroxide (NaOH) solution to straws (sprinkling) improves digestability and palatability of straws. It is added at the rate of 1 litre per kg of straw to remove lignin and harmful oxalates. Oxalates remove calcium in the form of calcium oxalate.

Silage making

Straw, along with some green grasses can be used for silage making during fodder scarcity.

Molasses

Molasses or brown sugar is a good source of energy to withstand severe winter. I use about 50–100 g of molasses, about 100 ml of edible oil and aobut 10 g of ginger powder per cattle to withstand stress of winter and also to make it act as an appetiser, to reduce dustiness of feed, and to provide unidentified nutrients like iron, etc. Maximum level of 15% should not be exceeded.

Oilseed cakes

Most oil cakes such as soya bean, groundnut, cotton seed, mustard, etc. are very good sources of protein (95% of nitrogen). Digestibility is also extremely good (75 to 95%). I have used these cakes to increase milk yield, milk fat percentage, and during late pregnancy. They also provide good amount of amino acids such as methionine, lysine and cystine. Beware of bad quality cakes with more than 10% moisture which can cause fungal toxicosis, particularly aflatoxin. Cotton seed cake is good to increase buffalo milk fat and yield but is poor in methionine, lysine and cystine. Expeller make cotton seed cakes contain 200–500 mg/kg of toxic gossypol. Hence judiciously use cotton seed cake. Soya bean meal or cake contains 44 to 49%

protein but they should be used only within limits to prevent bad effects of (a) goitrogenic substance, (b) trypsin inhibitor and (c) a plant estrogen.

Other good meals are Niger cake (MP, Maharashtra and AP). It is also rich in methionine and lysine. Guar meal (Gujarat, Rajasthan and MP); Neem cake which can be added below 15 to 20%.

Enhancing Rumen Performance (ERP)

Optimisation of energy enhances better return. In cows 12% of energy is wasted as methane (toxic gas). Neospark Drugs and Chemicals supply ERP liquid for this. It contains copper, cobalt, sulphur, and probiotics. It destroys pathogens and:
1. Stops production of methane.
2. Destroys harmful bacteria.
3. Probiotics support digestive bacteria and protozoa.
4. Cobalt helps B_{12} synthesis and propionate utilization.
5. Copper helps optimal rumen fermentation + propionate production.
6. Sulphur helps synthesis of amino acids, vitamins and enzymes.

All the above factors help in increasing quality and quantity of milk from cows and buffaloes.

Presentation

1. *ERP Liquid* (Neospark product).
   Dose: a. Regularly—100 ml/day/cow for 10 days in mouth (orally).
   b. Rumen problems: 100 ml twice daily for 3 to 5 days (orally).
   It can be diluted with equal quantity of water.
2. *Provisacc Forte* (Pfizer): It contains Amaferm, pH stabilisers, probiotics, and organic supplements as powder.
   Function: Improves fibre digestion, feed utilisation, milk quality and quantity.
   Presentation: 6 sachets of 20 g each.
   Dose: 1–2 sachets/day/animal, orally.
   Or 20–40 g/day/animal orally.
3. *Galac Shot (Cargil):* Contains glycogenic substances, bypass fat, herbal extracts. It improves milk quality and quantity.
   Presentation: 1 and 5 kg.
   Dose: 100 g/cow/day, orally.
4. *Rumisacc bolus* (Zydus): Contains amylase, cellulose, xylanase, papain, liver extract, ginger, methionins, sachromyces, L-lysine, histidine, leucine, lactobacillus, enzymes, amino acids, biostimulants and magnesium tricilicate, soya bean meal
   Dose: Cow 2–4 boli for 3–5 days, orally (packing of 30 strips of 4 bolus).
5. *Biobloom:* Saccharomyces sp, lactobacillus, phytase, cellulase, xylanase, pectinase, protein 50%, unknown growth factor, vitamins and minerals.
   Packing: 250 g and 1 kg.
   Dose: Cow, buffalo 15 g/day.
   Calf, goat, sheep 5 g/day.

Water for Cattle

It is important to understand that too hard water will seriously retard milk production and may indirectly kill calves by killing ruminal microflora. The result is impaction of rumen, alkaline indigestion, etc.

Requirement of drinking water

Body weight	Winter	Summer
50 kg	3.6 litres	5.3 litres
400 kg	35.2 litres	46.2 litres (heifers)
400 kg (cow) in milk	26.5 litres	270 litres

▪ IMPORTANT MINERALS

1. *Magnesium:* Deficiency results in:
   a. Marked vasodilatation and redness of skin.
   b. Twiching of muscles (especially of face).
   c. Staggering gait and ultimately, tetany.
2. *Iron*: For haemoglobin and myoglobin formation. Anaemia of cattle is the most prevalent malady of village cattle in India which goes undetected or uncared by field veterinarians.
3. *Zinc*: Zinc deficiency most commonly results in unhealthy skin, hairs, ringworm disease, loss of hairs (hirless parts), poor wound healing, and loss of appetite.
4. *Copper*: Deficiency causes 'enzootic ataxia' or 'paralytic hind legs' in lambs due to poor myelin synthesis. Abnormal (poor) hair colour, 'falling disease' in calves due to severe anaemia, diarrhoea (scouring disease) in cattle. In lambs there is dragging of lifeless legs called 'sway back'.
5. *Cobalt*: Cobalt is also deficient in green fodders like copper because the grasses, due to shortage in India are made to grow fast by using chemical fertilisers but minerals like copper, cobalt, etc. cannot keep pace with plant growth, resulting in deficiency in plants. I have observed good response in hundreds of calves kept among thousands of cattle kept in our branches of Surat Panjarapole by injecting copper and cobalt (self-made). In cobalt deficiency, the calves become weak ('wasting disease') or they have staggering gait ('enzootic marasmus'). They show watery discharge (tears) from eyes and nose. There may be frothy material outside lips. Such animals become recumbent and die.

Cobalt injections

Toxic dose of cobalt is 40–45 mg of elemental cobalt per kg BW per day. Use these injections with caution. They may not be used in private practice. These are mentioned only to convey my experience with discarded animals at Panjarapole.

I use injectable B complex containing mthylcobalamin injections (of Zydus). With 100 ml of Neuroxin-M. I dissolve 5 mg of cobaltous chloride hexahydrate extra pure (Hi Media; ref: RM673-100G) per 2 ml of the above. Then I mix 0.5 ml sterile ground nut oil (refined) per 2 ml. To this mixture some antibiotics are added in aseptic (laminar flow) cabin. 2 ml injection (5 mg Co) is injected at 5 to 8 days interval by SC route.

Copper Injections

Copper injections are made as above to contain 8 mg copper oxide AR (Hi Media, Ref no. GRM 732-100 C) per 2 ml of injectable B complex. This injection gave faster response in recombant calves. The calves stood up and slowly started moving about.

Legumes contain more cobalt than other green fodders. Liver etract injections such as 'Belamyl' and good feed mixtures should be given for quicker recovery. Liver contains more copper and cobalt than other tissues.

Supplemental Medication

Provisac Plus (Cargil, Provimi Animal Nutrition India): Contains in each bolus 50 mg copper sulphate, 20 mg cobalt sulphate besides zinc (100 mg), biotin, etc. It is given orally at the rate of 2 boli per day for 3 to 5 days.

Micro Power (Mineral liquid of Neospark): It contains, per 10 ml: Copper 15 mg; Cobalt 9 mg; Zinc 15 mg; Iodine 3.6 mg; Selenium 6 mg.
Dose: Cattle, etc. 15–30 ml per day.
   Calves, sheep, goats 5–10 ml per day.

Bexolive: Liquid by TTK Pharma
   It is also good and contains vitamins methionine, iron, copper, cobalt, selenium. Dose is almost as in case of 'Micro Power'. (Presentation 300 ml, 1 and 5 litres).

Co-Cu tablets: Contain copper and cobalt for oral feeding (packing of 50 tablets).
Dose: Cattle, etc. 4 tablets daily for 2–3 weeks.
   Sheep, goats 2 tablets daily for 2–3 weeks.

Chromium: Chromium is required for proper glucose and protein metabolism. It acts as a cofactor with insulin. It also reduces serum cholesterol level.

Manganese: Manganese as such does not produce typical symptoms in large animals but it is concerned with activation of several metabolic enzymes and calcification.

Chapter 18

Reproductive Disorders (Bovine)

In cows, the following reproductive disorders are important for which 'Provago' (Brihans Labs) provides a wide range of treatments.

■ COWS AND BUFFALOES

1. Anoestrus (silent or shy breeders).
2. Anovulatory heat or repeat breeders.
3. Follicular cyst (to be diagnosed by per rectum of ovarian palpation).
4. Luteal cyst (to be diagnosed by per rectal ovarian palpation).
5. Delayed ovulation.

Mares

1. Cystic ovaries—results in prolonged oestrum or short oestrus cycles
2. Anoestrus
3. Induced ovulation to synchronise with mating
   Pigs: Anoestrus
   Sheep and goats: Anoestrus
   Different reproductive disorders are summarised below as percentages of field cases.
   • 31.79% Anoestrus
   • 24.61% Repeat breeding
   • 14.35% Retention of placenta
   • 11.25% Abortion
   • 6.66% Pyometra
   • 5.12% Dystocia
   • 4.61% Endometritis
   • 1.53% Prolapse
   (M.H. Khan et al, 2016) Dystocia is outside the scope of this manual.

■ THREATENED ABORTION (COWS AND BUFFALOES)

1. *d-Pot (Injection IM)—Hydroxyprogestron (Zydus)*
   Habitual or threatened abortion—2 ml IM after 1.5 months of pregnancy; repeat 4–5 times after 10 days each.
   Repeat breeding: 1 ml IM after insemination. Repeat weekly for 3 weeks.
   Prolapse: 2 ml every 3rd day, if need be.
   Prolapse (Antepartum) 2 ml IM every 2 days × 3
2. *CRS (Zydus): Chelated Ranmix Shakti—rumen by pass:*
   Repeat breeding: 30 g per day total (1 kg or 2.5 kg pack) to be given for 10–15 days after AI (Contents: Zn, Cu, etc.).

Anoestrus: 30 g dose as above.

Threatened abortion: 30 g dose as above for repeat breeding.

3. *Cyclomin 7 (Zydus):* Cu, Co, iodine, iron, Mn, selenium and Zn; 7 minerals: For inducing natural heat, conception rate and involution of uterus in postparturient cows.

Natural heat: 1 bolus daily for 20 days.

Post AI: 8 days; 1 bolus daily (conception better).

Provago injection (marketed in India by Brihans Lab. Pvt. Ltd.)

Cows and buffaloes

Clinical signs	Conditions	Dose	Time of administration
No heat	Anoestrus	2.5 ml	On reporting. Inseminate on heat
Synchronisation of oestrus		2.5 ml	On start of scheduled plan
Repeating at regular interval	Anovulatory heat	5 ml	At heat. Inseminate in next heat
Prolonged heat	Follicular cyst	5 ml	At heat
Noheat (PCL)	Luteal cyst	5 ml	At heat
Repeating with advancing days	Ovulation	2.5 ml	At the time of insemination

Mares

Conditions	Dose
Cystic changes of the ovaries with or without prolonged permanent oestrus	10 ml
To induce ovulation of mature follicle and thereby to synchronize ovulation more closely with mating in mares	10 ml
Anoestrus	5 ml twice, with an interval of 24 hours

Swine

Condition	Dose
Anoestrus	2.5 ml

In sheep and goat

Condition	Dose
Anoestrus	1 ml

Can be given in all animals by IM or IV

Presentation: Vial of 2.5 ml with disposable syringe and swab.

Vial of 10 ml with 4 nos of disposable syringes and swabs.

50 g Minamil Gold given orally, daily, gives better results.

See also *Clostenol (Zydus)—Cloprostenol,* IM injection; dose 2 ml for oestrus induction, lutein cyst, metritis, pyometra, and synchronisation

For oestrus management in cattle give *Receptal (MSD Product)* 2.5 ml/5 ml. good for AI or natural service.

Hormone Products of MSD Animal Health Include

Receptal Vet

Composition	Indications	Dosage
Each ml contains Buserelin acetate 0.0042 mg	True anoestrus	5 ml, IM
	Improvement of conception rate (at the time of AI)	2.5 ml, IM
	Ovarian cyst (follicular), irregular oestrus, Nymphomania	5 ml, IM
	Delayed ovulation and anovulation	2.5 ml, IM
	Improvement of pregnancy rate (11–12 days post AI)	2.5 ml, IM
	Improvement of postpartum fertility (10–15 days postcalving)	5 ml, IM

Chorulon

Composition	Indications	Dosage	Presentation
Each vial contains human chorionic gonadotrophin (Hcg) as a white freeze-dried crystalline powder (1500 IU)	Improvement of conception rate (cows/ buffaloes)	1500 IU at AI or mating, IM or IV	Box containing 5 vials (1500 IU each) with 5 vials of solvent
	Enhancement of luteal function post AI	1500 IU, 4–6 days post AI, IM	
	Cystic ovarian disease (anoestrus, prolonged estrus, nymphomania)	3000 IV, IU	
	Induction of ovulation (mares)	1500–3000, IU, IM or IV, 24 hours before AI/mating	

Folligon

Composition	Indications	Dosage	Presentation
Each vial contains pregnant mare serum gonadotrophin (PMSG) as a freeze-dried crystalline powder (1000 IU)	*Females:* • Anoestrus • Super ovulation • Increase of fertility rate after progesterone pretreatment	Cow/buffalo Anoestrus: 500–1000 IU IM Super ovulation: 1500–3000 IU, IM between day 8–13 of cycle 300–700 IU, IM, at the end of a progestagen treatment	Box containing 5 vials (1000 IU each) with 5 vials of solvent

Crestar

Composition	Indications	Dosage	Presentation
Each application comprises: • One Crestar implant, containing 3.3 mg norgestomet for subcutaneous implantation in the outer face of the ear • Two ml crestar injection, containing 3 mg norgestomet and 5 mg oestradiol Valerate for intramuscular injection	Oestrus control in cattle (heifers and cows)	Day 0 = Crestar implant insertion + two ml Crestar injection IM Day 9 or day 10 = implant removal + PMSG 300 to 400 IU IM (if noncyclic) AI = dairy heifers: 48 hours after implant removal. *Dairy cows:* 56 hours after implant removal	25 sets (5 × 5'S) per box

Pregmate Injection

It contains cloprostenol, a synthetic prostaglandin. It causes regression of corpus luteum and onset of oestrus in 2 to 5 days.

Indications

1. To start oestrus and oestrus synchronisation.
2. It cures silent heat or subestrus.
3. It helps in chronic pyometra and chronic metritis by expulsion of pus or exudates.
4. It can expel mummified foetus (dead immature foetus).
5. It can be used for oestrus synchronisation (to get animals pregnant at desired time and delivery at desired time/season/month).

Dose and use

1. For luteolysis: Inject intramuscularly—2 ml
2. B. For abortion 1.5 ml (2 ml for animal above 455 kg)
   Without period: For milk—nil
                  For meat—1 day
   Presentation: 2 ml vial + syringe and needle.

Anoestrus and Repeat Breeding

1. Beta4vet (Hester product)
   It contains Beta-carotene, organic trace minerals and vitamin E.
   Indications: Anoestrus, repeat breeding, silent heat, abortions and retention of placenta
   Presentation: 1, 5, and 20 kg powder
   Dose: add 30 to 50 g daily in feed.
2. Zydabelin (Gonadorelin—synthetic gonadotrophin releasing hormone)
   Burselin acetate—0.0042 mg = Burselin 0.004 mg.

Indications

1. Improvement of conception rate of artificial insemination.
2. Infertility of ovarian defect.
3. Early induction of oestrus cycle after calving.
   Dose: Cattle and buffaloes: anoestrus—5 ml (IM, IV or SC route injection)
          Follicular cyst or nymphomania—2.5 ml
          Delayed ovulation—2.5 ml
          Improving results of AI—2.5 ml
   Mare: Anoestrus—5 ml twice after a 24 hour gap.

Purak Fertility Mixture (Tineta Pharma Pvt Ltd, Mumbai)

It contains traces of all minerals including cobalt, phosphorus, calcium, iron, etc. (10 minerals). Helps to bring animal to heat in cases of
1. Anoestrus suboestrus
2. Anaemia
   Dose: 30–35 g per animal/day or 1 kg/100 kg feed for oral feeding
   Packing: 1 kg and 10 kg.

Holler Bolus (Kepler Vet. Mission Pvt Ltd)

Like Purak mixture, this contains all the above minerals and also vitamin D_3-2000 IU, vitamin A-10000 IU and vitamin E 10 mg. Thus it is better than Purak.
Indications are as for Purak.

Dose: Anoestrus/silent heat—2 bolus twice daily. For treating mineral deficiency—2 bolus daily morning and evening.

Sajan Capsule

Each capsule contains Mrigakshi 600 mg, Tikshana 60 mg, Krishna pippali 60 mg and Sringavar 60 mg.

Indications: Nonspecific anoestrus, nonovulatory oestrus, and for inducing postpartum oestrus.

Dose: Cow, buffalo, heifer, mare—3 capsules/day.
Sheep, goat, bitches—2 capsules/day.
Packing: 6 capsule blister.

Janova (Ayurvet)

Contains Cittrullus colocynthis, Piper longum, and Piper nigram. Mimics action of FSH and LH.

Indications: Nonovulatory oestrus, repeat breeding, silent heat.

Dose: Cow, buffalo, mare 3 capsules/day for 2 days.
Ewes, doe, sow 2 capsules/day for 2 days.

■ RETENTION OF PLACENTA (ROP)

Retention of placenta is a common problem in all dairy units. It is essential to know the drugs which help to expel placenta and other uterine waste material. Such drugs are called ecbolic drugs.

1. *Expar (Ayurvet product)*
   Unique herbal preparation containing 3 herbal contents.
   Benefits
   a. Expulsion of placenta
   b. Involution (return to normal size) of uterus
   c. Expulsion of lochia (waste)
   d. Postpartum anoestrus is established
   Dosage: 100 ml liquid or 4 boli orally, twice daily—1st day
   50 ml liquid or 2 boli orally, twice daily—for next 3 days
   Packing: 500 ml bottle
   4 boli blister
2. *Metra* (Tineta Pharma Pvt Ltd, Mumbai)
   Herbal ecbolic containing 13 herbal constituents. Its uses are as described above. It also prevents uterine infection, pus formation and metritis.
   Dose: 75–100 ml daily in cows, etc.
   50 ml daily in small animals.
3. *Ergometrin (injection IV or IM).*

Uses:
  a. ROP treatment.
  b. Expulsion of lochia (waste of uterus).
  d. Reduces intercalving period.
  e. Reduces chanes of metritis and pyometra.
Dose: Cow, etc. 2–5 mg/animal IM/IV injection.
      Ewe, goat, etc. 0.5 to 1 mg/animal IM/IV injection.
Presentation: 5 ml vial (1 mg per ml) Zydus product.

4. *Utriplus* (Zydus product)
   Herbal drug containing 16 constituents of plants hence natural which works as cleanser/ecbolic.
   Indications:
     a. ROP
     b. Pyometra and metritis
     c. Easy postpartum heat
   Dose: Cow, etc. 100–125 ml orally
         Mare 50–75 ml orally
         Ewe, doe 20–40 ml orally

5. *Nexbolic* (Neovet, Intas)
   Methyl ergometrine injection (IM or IV). Dose as for Ergometrin.

6. *Himrop* (Himalaya)
   Herbal drug—see in the list of drugs.

▮ PROLAPSE OF UTERUS OR VAGINA

Prolapse of uterus is treated in three ways.

1. *Physically reducing the prolapsed part:* This is done with rubber gloves on hands. First inject IM xylazine 0–12 mg xylazine per 50 kg BW. See the effect 15–20 minutes later.
   If xylazine is not effective, then also inject 10 mg (1 ml) per 100 kg BW by IV or IM route. Desired painless condition develops in 5–15 minutes.
   Or

2. *Surgical:* If very severe stitches may have to be given to prevent prolapse.

3. *Hormonal:* After reduction of prolapse, hydroxy progesterone (P-Depot) 2–3 ml may be injected IM in cows or buffaloes after a few hours.

4. *Isoflud (Zydus)* may be injected (5–10 ml) by deep IM injection in cows and buffaloes to reduce inflammation.

5. *Neurovin M (Zydus):* May be injected at the rate of 5–10 ml IM/IV in large animals.

6. If fever develops, give antibiotic injection.

Homoeopathic

1. Give Cuprum met 30 1/2 teaspoonful in some water, 3 times a day (dextrose powder can be used for mixing.

2. Give colocynth 200 ¼ teaspoonful in dextrose powder.

Other drugs are:

1. *G plex bolus (Van Vet):* It is a herbal product. Give 4–6 bolus twice daily.
2. *Coaeg bolus (Van Vet):* To prevent much bleeding give 1–2 bolus twice daily.
3. *Phosphorus 200:* ½ teaspoonful in dextrose 2–3 times hourly will stop bleeding.
4. *Metricure IU (Zydus):* 30 and 100 ml povidone iodine and metronidazole to prevent uterine infections. Introduce 30–60 ml every 24 hours.
5. *Nexbolic (Intas) injection:* Contains methylergometrine. 5 ml vial. Dose for cattle and mare: 2–5 ml; small animals 0.5 to 1 ml IM or IV.
6. *Epidosin injection (TTK):* It is antispasmodic and painkiller. Injected IM at the dose rate of 10–15 ml.
7. *Spasmovet (Vetroquinol):* It is also antispasmodic containing dicyclomine hydrochloride to be used in all cases of prolapsed (vagina, vagina-cervix, uterus, urinary bladder, rectum, etc.). Prevents spasm of all these organs. Dose is 1 ml per 20 kg BW IM only. In sheep and goats, inject 1–2 ml; dogs 0.5 to 2 ml. If required, repeat after 12 hours.
8. Lignocain 8–10 ml may be injected in intervertebral space of top coccygeal vertebrae.

Chapter 19

Feeding Cattle and Buffaloes

▮ THUMB RULES

Thumb rules of feeding cattle and buffaloes:

- *Requirement for dry matter intake:* The requirement of the quantity of dry matter intake depends on the BW of the animal and also on the nature of its production. Cattle generally eat 2 to 2.5 kg of dry matter daily for every 100 kg BW. Buffaloes and crossbreed animals are heavier eaters and their dry matter consumption varies from 2.5 to 3 kg daily per 100 kg BW. The DM should be given as given below:

  Total dry matter:

  a. 1/3rd from concentrate.

  b. 2/3rd from roughage:

     i. 2/3rd from dry roughage or ¾ if sufficient legume is available.

     ii. 1/3rd from green fodder or ¼ if legumes are available.

- *Roughage and concentrate ratio:* In general, ration should contain 50% or more roughage and at least 17% crude fibre. Concentrate mix should be limited to no more than 50% or about 35% of the total ration dry matter.

  It is always economical to meet the animal's requirements from roughages as much as possible. The remaining portion can be met from concentrates. Concentrate mixture should be readymade cattle feed or home made and it should generally have:

  – 25–35% oilcakes

  – 10–25% cereal by products

  – 25–35% cereals/millets

  – 5–20% pulse husk

- *Maintenance Ration:* This is the minimum amount of feed required to maintain the essential body processes at their optimum rate without gain or loss in body weight or change in body composition. Under such circumstances compound concentrate mixture must be fed wich provides at least 20% protein (14–16% DCP) and 68–72% TDN.

- *Item for dairy cattle:* 1. Straw 4–6 kg

  2. Concentrate mixture 1–2 kg

- *Gestation Ration:* In the case of pregnancy, from fifth month onwards more nutrients should be provided for proper growth of foetus and to prepare the mother to produce more milk after calving. For this, in addition to maintenance ration, 1 to 2 kg of concentrate mixture is recommended.

- *Items for pregnant cow:* 1. Straw 5 kg or more

  2. Concentrate 1.5 + 2 kg

- *Production Ration:* Production ration is the additional quantity of ration for milk production over and above the maintenance requirement. For cows, 1 kg concentrate is required for every 2.5 kg of milk and for buffaloes 1 kg for every 2 kg of milk produced.
- *Item for milch cow:* 1. Straw 6 kg
    2. Concentrate mixture 7 kg (2 + 5 for 10 kg milk production).

Chapter 20

Food for Dogs and Cats

Summarised from the paper of V. Balakrishnan, Professor and Head, Animal Nutrition, Madras Veterinary College, Chennai.

Requirements of food ingredients in dogs and cats:

Nutrient	Dog	Cat
Protein	22%	28%
Fat	5%	9%
Calcium	1.1%	1%
Phosphorus	0.9%	0.8%
Iron (mg/kg BW)	60	100
Vitamin A (IU)	5000	1000
Zinc (mg/kg BW)	50	30
Vitamin D IU	500	1000
Vitamin B_1 mg	1	5
Choline mg	1200	2000

Sources

Meat: Meat contains 20–22% protein and 2–9% fat.

Milk and milk products: Milk, whey, cheese. This should not be included at high level. Lactose in milk is not so well-digested by canines.

Eggs: Eggs are a good source of most requirements. To avoid 'avidin', an antidigestive enzyme, it is better to feed boiled, or mildly fried egg to minimum of 1 egg a day. (Boiling or frying destroys avidin).

Cereals: Cereals contain about 12% moisture, 9–14% protein, 2–5% fat, and 70–80% carbohydrates. Cereals have enough B_1 and niacin, e.g. of cereals are wheat, rice, oats, and corn.

Fats and oils: Animal fats are palatable to dogs and cats as compared to vegetable and milk, fat, and butter.

Vegetables: Vegetables are rich in water and fibre. They may form small part of canines' foods in the form of potatoes, carrots, tomatoes, peas, beans, soya bean chunks, etc.

Biscuits: Dog biscuits may be fed as directed by the manufacturer.

Puppies: Puppies get enough nutrients from mothers' milk up to 4 weeks of life. Cow's milk is not a substitute for mother's milk. Cow's milk, if used, requires modification by canine specialist.

Feeding schedule for dogs:
- 3 weeks—small pieces of meat, or liver, or egg.
- 3 weeks to 3 months—4–5 times a day.

- 3–5 months—3 times a day.
- 5–10 months—2 times a day.
- Adult—once a day (maintenance).

  In mother's milk: More energy and protein twice a day

Single meal in adult has following advantages:
1. Large enough meal to give full satisfaction.
2. Underfeeding or overfeeding is less likely.
3. Time can be chosen to our convenience and defication within a few hours (at night) into two parts or 3 parts. Generally, feeding with family meal times results in obesity.

Average feeding rates:

Body weight	Dry matter
2.5–5 kg	3–3.5%
5–10 kg	2.5–3%
10 kg and more	2–2.5%

■ FEEDING CARE

1. Feeding by same person, same place, same time.
2. Remove leftover food within ½ to 1 hour.
3. Water should be always available.
4. No snack or sweets during meal.
5. Dog mother and pups should be fed separately.
6. Do not change food suddenly.
7. Clean feeding and water utensils daily.
8. Protein and fat digestibility is about 80–95%.

   Signs of inadequate nutrition are:
   a. Poor growth.
   b. Loss of weight.
   c. Reduction of haemoblobin and serum protein.
   d. Rough (not shining) hair coat.
   e. Limping movements and dullness.

■ HUMAN FOOD FOR DOGS

Family food (vegetarian) may be supplemented if necessary, by eggs or meat or milk or soya bean chunks.

Example of home-made dog food:

	Body weight		
	20 kg	25 kg	30 kg
Milk (ml)	150	200	250
Fish (g)	50	50	50
Mutton (g)	200	300	400
Rice (g, cooked)	100	150	150
Vitamin A, D₃, B complex	½ tablespoon	½ tablespoon	½ tablespoon
Bone meal	+	+	+
Iodised salt	2.5 g	2.5 g	2.5 g

- Dogs require 1.1% sodium and cats 0.5% sodium
- Taurine, an amino acid, is found mainly in meat
  Example of *home-made food for cat (adult)*
  - Liver 50 g
  - Milk 100 ml
  - Fish 50 g
  - Meat/chicken 150 g
  - Cooked rice 50 g
  - Vitamin A, D, B complex +
  - Minerals +
  - Iodised salt 1 g
  - Taurine +
- Cats are naturally carnivorous hence it is essential to add meat or liver in diet. Thiamine is essential for cats besides other vitamins. Omega 6 fatty acids and omega 3 fatty acids in the ratio of 5–10: 1 are essential for dogs and cats. Oils of safflower and corn are rich in these omegas.

Prebiotics and Probiotics

Probiotics and prebiotics are also desirable for dog and cat foods (health promoting microorganisms) example lactobacillus spp (at least traditional yoghurt 15–25 g a day may help to some extent). Commercial prebiotics and probiotics may be fed under the advise of a canine specialist.

Venkeys Pet Pvt Ltd of Pune supply dog and pet foods.

Cuddle Doggie 400 g pack: Contains 8% protein, 5% fat, and crude fiber 0.1%.

Cuddle Puppie: 400 g pack contains 8.5% protein, 6.5% fat, 0.7% crude fiber and 0.9% calcium and 0.7% phosphorus.

Shiv Cat: 400 g and 2 kg packs contain fish, poultry meat, corn, sunflower oil, Ca, phosphorus and vitamins for cats of 1 year or more age.

Other dogs and cat meals made by Venkys Pets are listed below. Follow the directions given with packing.

Regal Pup: 400 g, 4 kg, 15 kg packs; good for large breeds.

Regal meal: 400 g, 4 kg, 15 kg packs. Contains protein 20%, fat 10% and metabolic energy 3750 k cal/kg. It is a balanced food for all breeds.

Best in Show: 500 g, 4 kg, 15 kg packs for small and medium breeds.

Best in Show Puppy Starter: 1 kg pack.

Gutwell: Prebiotic and probiotic: feed 2–5 g twice a day.

Ven Cal Tab (package of 60 tabs): Give 1 to 4 tabs depending on size.

Cani-Care Forte (Vesper Pharma): To reduce obesity.

Commercial Food Products for Pets

Royal Canin

It is also available through some veterinary doctors. Different makes of it are available for different problems, e.g.

1. Acute pancreatitis—low fat, dry wet.

2. Ascites—cardiac, hepatic problem.
3. Convalescence—recovery after disease.
4. Gastrointestinal (low fat).
5. Hepatic—liver disease.
6. Hypoallergic—in allergic conditions.
7. Renal—kidney diseases.
8. Satiety.
9. Skin support.
10. Urinary.
11. Weight control.
    Consult veterinary doctor for advice.

Petz Home Food Plus (Zydus)

It is a complete balanced cereal mix (rice, wheat, soya bean, milk proteins, minerals (10 minerals), vitamins (9), choline, taurine, lysine, methionin (amino acids).

Indications

1. Complements home-made food for alround growth, pregnancy, nursing (28 nutrients).
2. Taurine helps in preventing dilatations of heart.
3. Improves immunity, dental health.
4. Easy to feed and 100% vegetarian.
   Dose: Growing pups 1 spoon (10 g) daily.
   Adult (maintenance) 2 spoons (20 g) daily.
   Pregnant and nursing 3 spoons (30 g) daily.
   Double dose for large and giant dogs.
   Presentation: 250 g.

Other Zydus Dog Foods

1. Canidine: For adult large and giant dogs in 1, 3, 10, and 15 kg.
2. Canidine: For small and medium dogs in 1, 3, 10, and 15 kg.
3. Canidine Puppy: Large and giant in 1, 3, 10, and 15 kg.
4. Canidine: For small and medium puppies in 1, 3, 10, and 15 kg.
   Made in Belgium (as claimed by Zydus).

Hairfall, Dandruff free, Allergy Free Food

Soft Coat (Vetina, *www.vetina.com*) Give orally or mix in food of dogs/cats at the rate of 0.5 ml/kg BW/day. (Multimolecular, mineral, vitamins, and micronutrients).

Royal Canine Products (Food)

Diet Canine	SKU (in kg)
Dry anallergenic	3
Dry anallergenic	8
Wet cardiac	0.41
Dry cardiac	2

Contd...

Diet Canine	SKU (in kg)
Wet convalescence	0.41
Dry diabetic	1.5
Wet gastrointestinal low fat	0.41
Dry gastrointestinal low fat	1.5
Wet gastrointestinal	0.40
Dry gastrointestinal	2
Wet hepatic	0.42
Dry hepatic	6
Dry hypoallergenic	2
Dry hypoallergenic	7
Dry mobility C2P	2
Dry mobility C2P+	7
Wet renal	0.41
Dry renal	2
Dry renal	7
Wet satiety	0.41
Dry satiety	1.5
Dry satiety	6
Dry satiety	12
Dry skin support	2
Wet urinary	0.41
Dry urinary	2
Dry weight control	1.5
Diet canine and feline	
Wet recovery can	0.195
Diet feline	
Wet renal (12 pouches)	1.02
Dry renal	2
Dry satiety	1.5
Dry satiety	3.5
Wet urinary (12 pouches)	1.2
Dry urinary	1.5
Wet sensitivity chicken (12 pouches)	1.2

Canine Diet Recommendations (Dry/Wet)

Oxalate kidney stones	Renal	Dry
	Renal	Wet
	Urinary s/o	Dry
	Urinary s/o	Wet
Poor appetite	Convalescent	Wet
	Gastrointestinal	Wet
	Recovery	Wet
Neoplasia (tumour/cancer)	Convalescent	Wet
	Gastrointestinal	Wet
Pre- /post-surgery	Recovery	Wet
Kidney failure	Renal	Wet Dry
Stress	Gastrointestinal	Dry Wet
Vomiting	Gastrointestinal	Dry
Gastrointestinal		Wet
Obesity	Weight control + diabetic support	Dry

'PEDIGREE' FOODS FOR PETS

Different types of food packs are available from Pedigree:
1. Pedigree adult vegetarian 100 g packet.
2. Pedigree puppy milk vegetarian 1.2 kg pack.
3. Pedigree veg 1.2 kg and 3 kg packets.

COMMON PET SUPPORTS

1. Pet Cal B_{12} liquid syrup—calcium and vitamin supplement (Zydus product).
2. PetoLiv syrup—200 ml liquid—liver tonic (Ek Tek pharma).
3. Petovit multi drops—multivitamin drops, 30 ml (Ek Tek Pharma).
4. Petovit syrup 200 ml (Ek Tek Pharma).
5. Petocoat syrup, 200 ml (Ek Tek Pharma) for shining body coat.
6. Pet Kuff syrup, 100 ml (Ek Tek Pharma).
7. Pet joint tablets, 12 or 100 tabs, for joint problems (Pet Care product).
8. Pet Derm shampoo, 200 ml, Zoetis product.
9. Peto vate ointment 20 g, for injuries and infections (Ek Tek Pharma).
10. Probisk biscuits, 400 g (Mera Pet product).
11. Procott biscuits, 400 g (Mera Pet product).
12. Prolifur soup, 3 in 1, 100 g (Mera Pet product).
13. Pet-O-Ease syrup, 100 ml (Ek Tek Pharma).

Pedigree daily feeding guide of adult, 100% vegetarian, dry			
Adult body weight	Breeds	Recommended daily food amount(g)	
Small up to 10 kg, 7–9 months	Miniature Pomerian	110–140	Manufactured by
	Pug, Tibetian	130–170	Huhtamaki-PPL Ltd
	Spaniel, Lhasa Apso, terriers	146–170	Hyderabad
Medium 10–25 kg, 9–12 months	Duschund	170–12	Complete balanced food
	Crossbred	190–260	by Pedigree
	Indian pom.	220–240	
	Cocker spaniel	260–320	
	Beagle	280–310	
Large, 25–50 kg, 12–18 months	Boxer	34–410	Pedigree India, phone:
	Cross bred	340–430	1800407112121,
	Retriever	370–450	918452306691
	Dalmatian	390–450	
	Labrador	390–470	
	Doberman, Ger Shephard	410–500	
Giant, 50–100 kg	Great dane	560–650	
	St. Bernard	770–900	
	Mastiff	860–990	

HOME FOOD PLUS (Zydus Product)

It is a dog food supplement not complete food. It contains cereal mix, malt, vegetable fat, caramel, sugar, lactic acid and bacteria.

Uses

It is used in addition to home food for proper development of teeth, bones, hair coat and general health care.

Dosage: 250 g packing is available.

For growing pups 1 spoon (10 g) twice daily.

Adult dogs 2 spoons (20 g), twice daily.

Pregnant and nursing bitches 3 spoonfuls, twice a day.

Caldipet (Zydus)

A tonic. Give 10 ml orally, twice a day; puppies 5 ml.

Or **Verol (Zydus) syrup**—same dose as caldipet.

Milk O Pet (Weaning) in 400 g box packing.

Contains protein, fat, carbohydrates, all minerals, vitamins and amino acids. It is a puppy weaning formula with adequate nutrition. It is mixed with water for serving.

Dose

Age	Quantity per serving (g)	Water (ml)	Number of daily servings
Till 4 weeks	10–20	50–60	4–5
4–8 weeks	20–25	60–70	3–4
Above 8 weeks	25–30	75–90	2–3

Serelac—weaning formula for weaning pups and kittens (Vetina Co), dose as above

■ TOP CAT (PFIZER ANIMAL HEALTH)

Complete nutrition for cats.

Features

1. High protein (10%) to ensure strong muscles.
2. Omega 6 and 3 for health, body coat, and skin.
3. Probiotic and Yucca extracts.
4. Vitamins, taurine, methionine, linoleic acid, calcium, spongenin, lysine, and phosphorus.

   Presentation: 1, 2, and 10 kg packs.

   Dose: Start feeding after 30 days of age. Feed as per directions gien on the packet.

Saborvidha (Pfizer): Complete food for dogs.

Canobits (Pfizer): Complete food for dogs. Use both these products as per directions given on packets.

Chapter 21

Mineral Supplements (Ruminants) for Large Animals

Mineral supplements are essential to manage the following conditions:
1. Anoestrus, silent heat, repeat breeding.
2. Improve conception/fertility.
3. Reproductive health.
4. Growth of calves and heifers.
5. Prevent deficiency diseases and anorexia.
6. Proper ruminal microflora/digestion.
7. Provide bypass minerals, proteins, and fats.
8. Selenium is most important for antioxidant defence and late pregnancy.
9. Deficiency diseases, such as milk fever, bone diseases, skin diseases, anaemia, metabolic diseases, falling disease, enzootic marasmus.
10. Maintain or improve milk yield.
11. Improve/maintain immune system (most important is zinc for B and T cell defence. Copper is essential for killing of bacteria by leucocytes.
12. Postparturient problems (calving problems).

Examples:
1. *CRS (Zydus product):* It is an excellent product having zinc (9600 mg), copper (4500 mg), cobalt (112.6 mg), iodine (375 mg), selenium (7.5 mg), magnesium (4500 mg), potassium (75 mg), sodium (4500 mg), sulphur (5400 mg), calcium (191.25 g), phosphorus (95.62 g), vitamin A (525000 IU), vitamin D_3 (52500 IU), vitamin E (187.5 mg), vitamin B_3 (750 mg), biotin (500 mg), methionine (94.2 g). It is best for high yielding cows and buffaloes.
   Dose: 30 g/day/animal (cows).
   Packing: 1 kg and 2.5 kg.
   Minerals are chelated hence best bioavailable.
2. *Best Min (Cargil product):* Almost similar contents as CRS (Nonchelated) and probably lesser quantity.
   Dose: Cow, etc. 100–200 g/day.
         Calf, sheep, etc. 50–75 g/day.
3. *Hi FCR powder (Hester):* Contains monensin, biotin, choline, minerals and metabolites.
   Packing: 100 g
   Dose: 10 g daily for 10 days (cows).
4. *Profimin Forte (Vets Pharma).*
5. *Nutricell powder (TTK Healthcare):* Similar to CRS powder. It is chelated. It also has chromium and nicotinamide.

6. *VM powder (MSD product):* Contains 12 important minerals and chromium almost as in CRS.
   Packing: 1, 5, 25 kg; Dose: as for CSR.
7. *Holler (Kepler):* Contains Ca, Zn, Fe, Se, Cu, Co (chelated).
8. *Utramin (Neospark):* Contains almost all minerals, DL methionine, and L-Lysine.
   Dose: cows, etc: 50 g day/animal; calves, sheep, goats, etc. 25–30 g/day orally.
9. *Totavit Strong (Vets Mankind product):* Methochelated, contains 12 minerals, 5 vitamins, 2 amino acids and 2 probiotics.
   Dose: Cows, etc. 30–50 g/day/animal.
      Small animals 15–20 g /day/animal.
10. *Minfa Strong* (Bovicura/Intas): Contains 12 minerals and vitamins A, D_3, and E.
    Dose: Cow, etc. 50 g/day/animal.
       Calf: 20 g.
    Package: 1, 3, and 5 kg.
11. *Lykamin powder* (Lyka/Alovera product): Contains 8 minerals and 2 amino acids
    Dose: Cow, etc. 30 g/day/animal.
       Calf, goat, etc. 10 g/day/animal.
12. *Minamil* (Brihans Lab): Contains 9 minerals, 9 vitamins including choline in powder form.
    Dose: Cows, etc. 20–25 g/animal/day.
       Calf and goats, etc. 5–10 g/day/animal.
    Poultry: 20–50 g/100 birds.
    Package: 250 g, 1, 6, 25, and 30 kg.
13. *Agrimin powder* (Virbac product): Contains 12 minerals, methionine and Lysine.
    Dose: Cows, etc. 50 g/day/animal.
       Small animals 10–15 g/day/animal.
    Packing: 1 and 10 kg.
14. Agrimin Forte: Also contains A, D_3, E and minerals extra.
    Dose: as above (Agrimin).
    Packing: 1 and 10 kg.
15. Chelated Agrimin Forte: Chelated minerals as in Agrimin powder.
    Dose: as for item 13 and 14 above.
    Packing: 0.5, 1 and 5 kg.
16. *Bovimin-B:* Contains chelated minerals, nickel and chromium.
    Dose: Cows, etc. 40 g/day/animal.
       Small animals: 20 g/day/animal.
    Package: 1.2, 6, and 24 kg.
17. Alvite-M (Alembic): Contains chelated minerals.
    Dose as for Minamil.
    Packing: 1, 5, and 25 kg.

■ HEAT MANAGEMENT

Hot summer may pose great problems for cows, buffaloes and sheep. Humidity may add additional stress in milk, eggs, and wool production in animals and also in their young ones. The problem has been magnified by global warming and dwindling soft water resources and deforestation (Fig. 21.1).

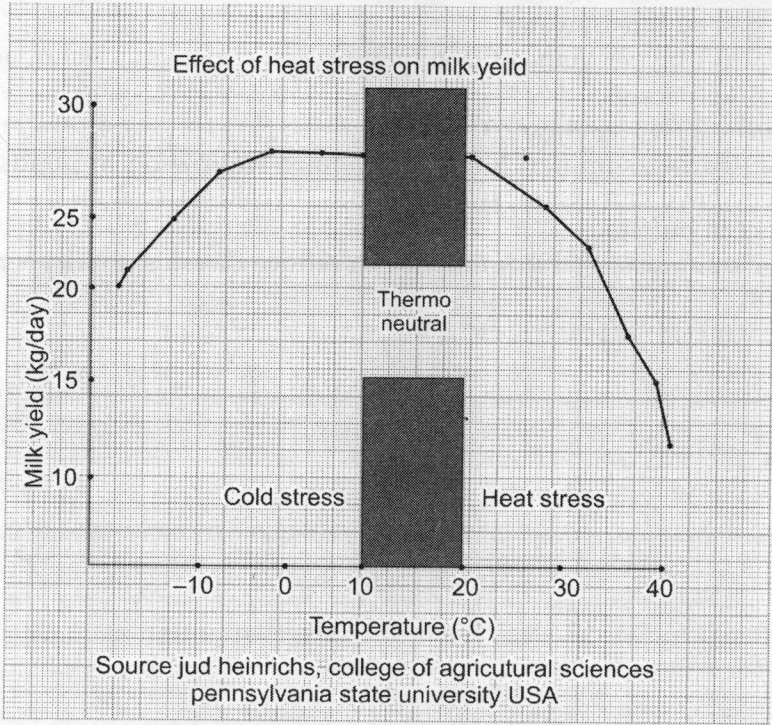

Fig. 21.1: Heat management

Measures

1. As much plantation around the house as possible.
2. In poultry, foggers are used to spray water fumes to reduce warmth and prevent heat stroke.
3. Amount of vitamin C may be increased to much more than normal without any harmful effect.
4. Replina (oral powder by TTK) is an antiheat stress product for poultry but I have used it to reduce mortality in summer in cow and buffalo calves in Surat which remains hot and humid in hot months of May and June.

Contents

1. Sodium salicylate—reduces level of catecholamines during heat stress.
2. Glycine and protein hydrolysate: reduces stress of low protein due to less food intake.
3. Sodium bicarbonate—prevents excessive acidosis due to catabolism.
4. Sodium citrate—corrects acid base balance.
5. Magnesium chloride—stops stress-induced oxidative damages.
6. Sodium and potassium chlorides and calcium lactate—help to reduce metabolic heat production.
7. *Vitamin C:* It is an antioxidant which prevents formation of free radicals which eliminate metabolic toxins. Available as ascorbic acid injections of Juggat Pharma.

Dosage: 1 g per 2 litre of water.

0.5 to 1 kg per tonne of feed (poultry)

Packaging: 1 kg packets.

Manufacturers: TTK Healthcare, Chennai.

Wallowing: During summer, buffaloes require wallowing in ponds or rivers because they have hardly any sweat glands. Thyroid-adrenal mechanism is also less efficient in buffaloes.

Supportive treatment: *Nervech injection* to reduce convulsions, hyperaesthesia, and tremor.

Cow, etc. 10 ml IM/IV; calves, etc. 1 to 2 ml.

Chapter 22

Miscellaneous Health Problems

ACUTE VIRAL HEPATITIS

It may or may not be with jaundice. Treatment should be continued till serum bilirubin returns to <1.5 mg/100 ml.

Hospitalise the dog if there is:
1. Persistant vomiting.
2. Prolonged fever.
3. Disturbed sleep.
4. If signs of ascites are seen, it indicates advanced stage.

Food

If appetite is good, continue normal food but not high protein and fat (oily) food. If possible, give Royal Canin Hepatic dry or wet food. For cats, give Top Cat (Pfizer) or Home Food Plus (Zydus).

Treatment

1. If there is fever, give antipyretics (*Melonex P*, *Vetalgin*, *FevNil*, etc.).
2. *Broton Vet* (liver tonic of Virbac 10 ml daily for 5 days.
3. *Vet DMG 125 liquid (Vetina Distributors LLP, Pune):* Presentation of 30 ml which acts as immunity support system, improves liver metabolism.
   Dose: Give following dose twice daily, orally for 2 weeks:

   Dogs/cats
   – Up to 5 kg: 0.25 ml.
   – 5–10 kg: 0.5 ml.
   – 20–35 kg: 1.5 ml.
   – Over 45 kg: 3 ml.
4. *Liv 52 (Himalayas) drops:* Give 7–8 drops morning and evening daily.
5. *Liverolin:* Pet syrup (Zydus) herbal product.
   Presentation: 150 ml.
   Dose: Up to 5 kg 1/2 teaspoonful, 2–3 times a day.
   5–15 kg: 1 teaspoonful, 2–3 times a day.
6. *Tefroli syrup (TTK):* It is a herbal syrup, hepatoprotective, appetiser, and immuno-stimulant
   Dose: Dogs and cats: 5–10 ml daily.
   Cattle: 10–20 ml daily.

Homoeopathic

Jondila syrup (Medisynth)—use as directed by the manufacturer.

For recovery phase

Totavit Strong (Mankind): It contains 5 vitamins, 12 minerals, 2 amino acids, and 2 *probiotics in banana flavour.*

Dose: 15–20 g with food or milk

■ ANOREXIA (LOSS OF APPETITE)

1. *Hepaways (Mankind):* Presentation of 500 ml, 200 ml, 1 litre.
   Dose: Dogs/cats 5–10 ml daily.
           Large animals 40 ml daily.
2. *BoviLax (Neospark) powder:* Corrects anorexia, inappetance, detoxifies and is a laxative.
   Dose: Cattle, etc. 250 g/day.
           Calves, sheep, goat 60 g/day.
3. *Amyst Bolus (Tineta):* Contains Saccharomyces, Asp oryzae and sea flora.
   Indications: Anorexia, acidosis, dyspepsia.
   Dose: Large animals 1–2 bolus; small animals 1/2 to 1 bolus twice a day.
   Packing: 30 × 2 boli.
4. *Feed Well gel (Neospark):* Feed 1 tube of gel (250 ml) per day.

Homoeopathic

Pulsatilla 200: Pets 2–3 drops in sugar pills, 2–3 times a day. It is excellent.

■ XYLAZINE (PRODUCT OF G. LOUCATOS, MUMBAI)

Description

Xylazine is a sedative, anaesthetic and muscle relaxant. Ruminants are the most sensitive of the domestic animals to action of Xylazine. In cattle and buffaloes, dose that produce deep sedation and analgesia is one tenth of the dose required in horses, dogs, cats, etc. Aged or sick bovines that have undergone severe physical exertion are found to respond more strongly to Xylazine.

Composition

Each ml of Xylazine injection contains Xylazine Hydrochloride B.Vet.C. 23.32 mg equivalent to Xylazine 20 mg.

Indications

Xylazine is for sedation, analgesia, anaesthesia, and muscle relaxation.
   Administration: Intramuscular route.
   Dosage: Cattle and buffaloes.
   Dose level I: 0.12 ml/50 kg 0.25 ml/100 kg.
                   1.20 ml/500 kg is given for the following purpose:
1. Tranqualize the animal, load in a vehicle and let it get accustomed to new surroundings.
2. Complete weighing and dressing.

3. Artificial insemination, e.g. ferocious animals like Khillari, Kankrej, Tharparkar breeds.
4. Prolaps of uterus.
5. Correction of torsion of uterus.
6. Ruminotomy.
7. Caesarean.

Dose level II: 0.25 ml/50 kg.
               0.50 ml/100 kg.
               2.50 ml/500 kg.
1. Minor surgical operation of teats.
2. Obstruction of the oesophagus.
3. Insertion of nose ring.

Dose Level III: 0.50 ml/50 kg.
               1.00 ml/100 kg.
               5.00 ml/500 kg.
(combined with local anaesthesia)
1. Major operation dehorning.
2. Castration.
3. Vasectomy.

Dose Level IV: 0.75 ml/50 kg.
               1.50 ml/100 kg.
               7.50 ml/500 kg.
For undomesticated animals for prolonged operations. Several hours of fasting is required.

Horse dosage: 5–10 ml/100 kg BW (equivalent to 100–200 mg/100 kg BW). Deep sedation with an individually variable degree of analgesia and distinct muscle relaxation, adequate for (1) loading, (2) shoeing, (3) examinations, (4) treatment of wounds and (5) obstetrical interference.

Precaution in cattle, buffalo and horse: The tympany that may occur in any ruminant should be relieved by placing the animals in sternal recumbency. To prevent the aspiration of saliva or food material, the head and the neck should be lowered. Animals should be fasted before the administration of high doses. The drug should not be used during the last month of pregnancy in view of the possibility of premature birth. When the subsequent period of hypnosis is prolonged, the animal should be protected against chilling or overexposure to direct sunlight. Caution is required in pulmonary conditions. In accidental overdoses, artificial respiration and central analeptics should be used.

Sheep dosage: 0.5 ml/25 kg BW. Pig dosage is 1.0 ml/33 kg BW.

Dog dosage: 0.5 to 1.5 ml/10 kg BW (equivalent to 10–30 mg/10 kg BW). The effect is adequate for procedures that are not associated with considerable degree of pain, such as:
1. Dressing.
2. Scaling of teeth.
3. Treatment of otitis.
4. Wounds, etc.

Cat dosage: 0.05 –0.1 ml/1 kg BW (equivalent to 1–2 mg/kg BW) the effect is adequate for procedures that are not associated with any considerable degree of pain such as:
1. Clinical and radiographical examination.
2. Scaling of teeth.
3. Treatment of dressing of wounds.
4. Induction of local or general anaesthesia.

For painful conditions of dog and cat: Required dose of Xylazine with atropine medication to reduce vagal activity. Barbiturate dose to be reduced to about 1/3 to 1/4.

Contraindications in dog and cat: Xylazine should not be used in obstruction of oesophagus, torsion of the stomach, hernia, etc. Caution is required in pulmonary condition.

Special caution on use of Xylazine in dogs and cats: When the stomach is full, vomiting occurs before the development of the effect. The vomiting stimulus can be considerably reduced by fasting for 6 to 24 hours.

Other domestic species/zoo and wild animals: Based on pharmacological properties, Xylazine injection can be used in other domestic species, zoo and wild animals. It is usually injected by intramuscular route, the onset of action is within 3–5 minutes and is augmented up to 15 minutes post injection after which the animals are usually approached.

■ MIND CALMING TABLETS (VETINA DISTRIBUTORS, PUNE)

Contents
1. Extract of chamomile—A proven stress remover.
2. Ginger—Anxiolytic and 5-HT$_3$ antagonist.
3. Velerian—produces enzymes which breakdown GABA.

Indications
1. Separation from place, society, or house.
2. Travelling stress.
3. During fireworks, excessive barking, aggression.
4. Violent behaviour.
    Dose: Up to 5 kg 1 tablet/day.
         5–10 kg 2 tablets.
         10–15 kg 3 tablets.
         15 kg and above 4 tablets.
    Packing: 30 tablets.

■ ALLERGY AND HYPERSENSITIVITY

Increased reactivity of animal tissues to an antigen (foreign substance) is called allergy or hypersensitivity.

Type I: Reaction of allergen or antigen with antibodies already present in blood or fixed to some cells. The antigen-antibody reaction produces a chain of biochemicals which cause contraction of smooth muscles resulting in:

1. Increased capillary permeability such as urticaria, itching, swelling in skin and inflammation
2. Immunological reaction without release of biochemical mediators. Results are anaemia, glomerulonephritis, serum sickness.

Type II: Autoimmune diseases such as haemolytic anaemia (wrong blood transfusion) thrombocytic purpura as in viral infections of dogs.

Type III: Arthus type reaction. This type of reaction occurs in previously sensitised animal after intradermal entry of any antigen. The antigen antibodies precipitate in the form of complex, attract and complement or products attract neutrophils and release lysosomal enzymes from damaged cells which produce inflammation.

Type IV: Cell-mediated or delayed hypersensitivity reactions, e.g. mycoplasmal pneumonia, tuberculin reaction.
Among animals type I is more often seen and brought for treatment.

Treatment

Most of the problems are brought as urticarial patches in skin not responding to antifungal and ectoparasitic treatment.

1. *Trellergin injection (Treffer Pharma):* Chlorpheniramine maleate; 30 ml vial.
   Dose: Large animals 3–5 ml; small animals 0.5–1 ml by IM injection.
2. *Wysolon tablets* 10 mg may be given to a dog at the rate of 0.5 mg/kg BW for only a few days.
3. *Avil*: Tablet at the rate of 1 mg per kg BW for a few days.
4. *Isoflud (Zydus) injection*: Cattle 5–10 ml IM injection.
5. *Bovistamin injection* (Bovian Health Care): Chlorpheniramine maleate injection 30 ml and 100 ml.
   Dose: 1 ml/20 kg BW by IM route only.
6. *Avil injection* (Hoechst)—same use as above, no. 5.
7. *Chlorazin (Zydus)*: Dose—Cow, etc. 3–5 ml IM once a day; dogs—0.5–2 ml IM injection.
8. *Allergia tablets for dogs* (Vetina Distributors, Pune).

Homoeopathic

Homoeopathic drugs may give safe and lasting treatment.
Apis mel 30 or 200: 10–20 globules may be given 3 times a day or more frequently in acute case.
Arsenicum album 30: May be given twice daily for more prolonged treatment.
Urtica urens 30: May be given along with above 2 drugs.

■ CHRONIC DIARRHOEA (DOGS) (Fig. 22.1)

Steps

1. Rule out the presence of intestinal worms.
2. Take body temperature to rule out fever/infection.
3. Enquire about food given and stop raw vegetable (tomatoes, etc.) intake, too much heavy diet (fat, eggs, meat, cheese, etc).

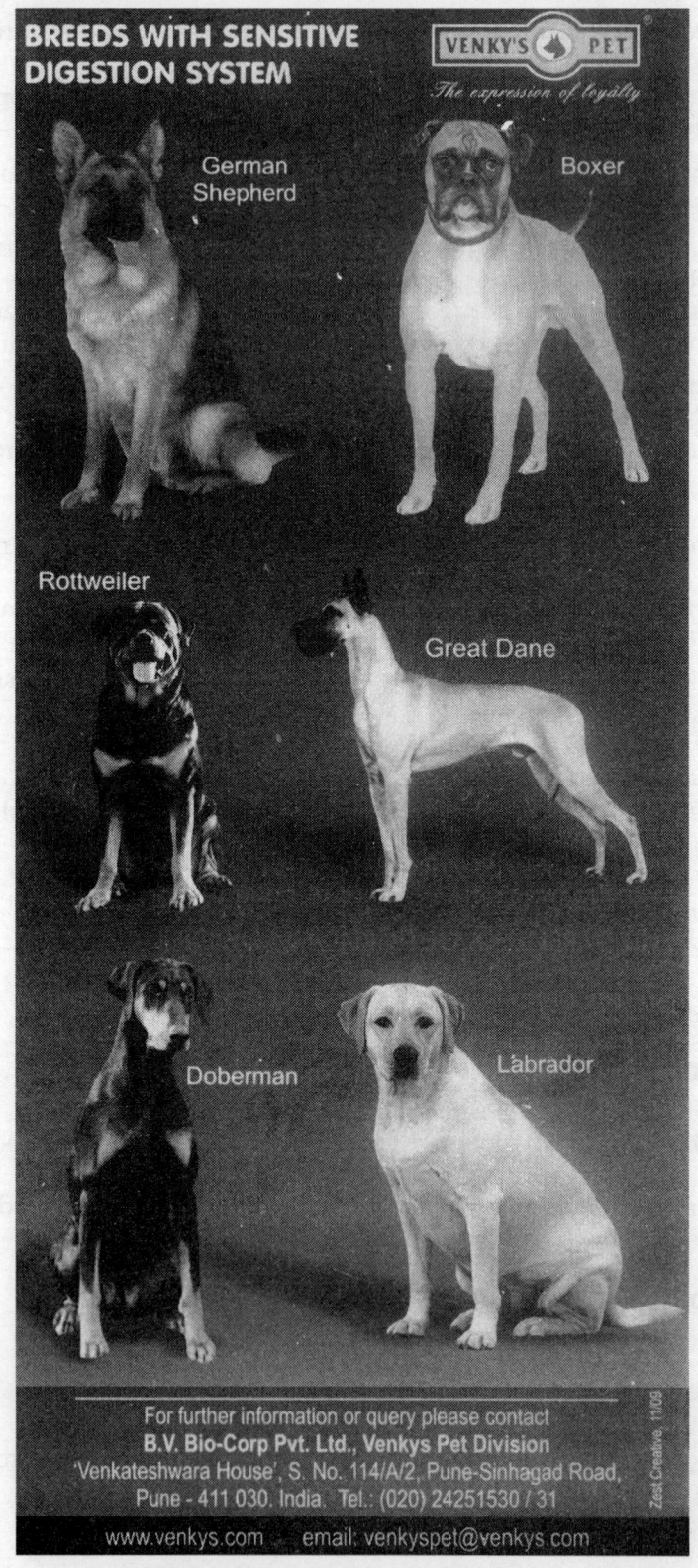

Fig. 22.1: Chronic diarrhoea (dogs)

Give

1. *Ipakitine Feed Supplement* (Vetoqinol), presentation of 180 g powder according to BW. Dosage: 3–5 kg, 2 scoops; 10 kg, 4 scoops; 15 kg, 6 scoops; 20 kg, 8 scoops.
2. *Cypon syrup*: Contains appetisers, choline and sorbitol.
   Dose: ¼, ½ teaspoonfuls once or twice a day.
3. *Give 9 kinds of biochemic mixture* given earlier, about ½ teaspoonful, dissolved in 6–8 teaspoonful warm water. Start with 1 teaspoonful (orally) then ½ teaspoonful hourly or 2 hourly/daily till recovery.
4. Tablet B complex- Becom L or Becozinc 1 daily.
5. If parasites are suspected, give: Parazisam Plus (Vetoquinol). For all round-worms, whipworms, hookworms (blood suckers) and hydatid worms—1 tablet/10 kg BW.
6. If fever, give Meriquin (Enrofloxacin) of Vetoquinol Co., presentation of 10 tablet strip of 50 and 150 mg.
   Dose for dog/cat: 5 mg/kg BW for 5 days. In severe cases, extend for 7–10 days.
7. Unienzyme tablets: 1 tablet after meals.

OEDEMA

Oedema means accumulation of watery fluid of noninflammatory origin anywhere in the body. Treatment can be done by Ridema.
   Ridema contains Frusemide 50 mg per ml (Vetoquinol product). Oedema of any type including oedema of udder in cows, etc.
   Dose: Cattle and buffaloes: 0.5 to 1.0 mg/kg BW by IM injection.
      Horse: 0.5–1 mg/kg/ daily IM 2 times a day.
      Dog/cat: 2.5 to 5 mg/kg BW or 2 times a day IM or IV.
   Presentation: 10 ml.
   Serakind Plus (Mankind): Serraptioreptidase enzyme + paracetamol bolus
   Indications: Swollen and painful udder, oedema, yolk gall, abscess, oedema anywhere.
   Dose: Large animals—2 bolus daily for 3–5 days, orally.
      Small animals—1 bolus daily for 3–5 days.

HOOF DISORDERS

Lameness, hoof deformities, slow healing of wounds may be treated by organic zinc (Fig. 22.2)

Treatment: Glymet—Zinc 22% (product of Merial Animal Health), presentation of 100 g powder

Dose: Cattle, etc. 2 g/day in feed.
      Or 200 g/tonne of feed.
   It is also useful for treatment of Degnala disease, chronic skin diseases, lameness, FMD, PPR (feet), foot rot in sheep and goats.

Homoeopathic: Calendula ointment and Calendula Q, 1/4 teaspoonful orally BD.

DIARRHOEA AND DYSENTERY OF UNKNOWN ORIGIN

Sometimes, diarrhoea and dysentery may not respond to usual treatment. In such cases:
1. *Rocklow* (a bolus of Kepler Vet Mission Pvt Ltd) may be tried. It contains Ofloxacin 1000 mg and Ornidazoe 1800 mg.

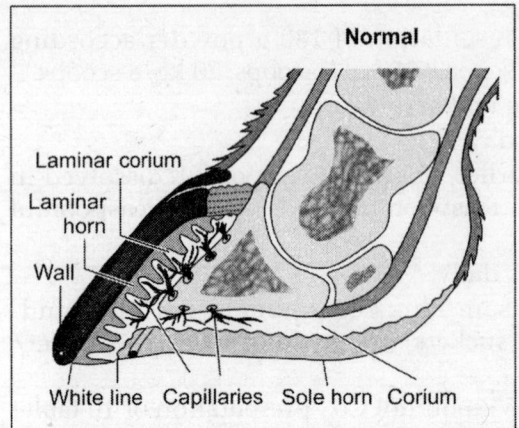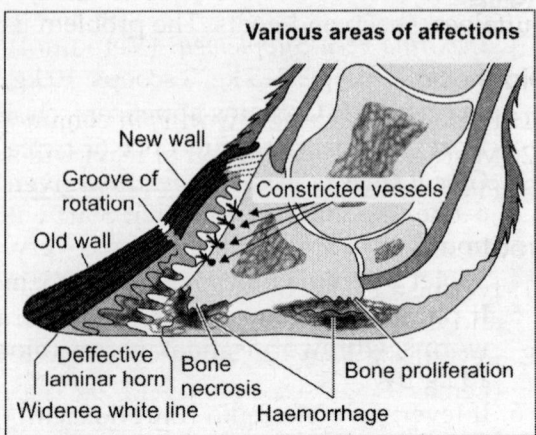

Fig. 22.2: Hoof deformities

Dose: Cattle and buffaloes: 1 bolus per 100 kg or 3 boli for 300 kg BW orally in jaggary or molasses for 3 to 5 days. Ofloxacin inhibits DNA gyrass necessary to hold bacterial DNA helix hence bacteria get killed.

2. *ORT Calf* (like ORS; Carus Labs, New Delhi): Mix A and B sachets in 1 litre water, feed 2–3 times a day.

■ COLIC

Occasionally animals show signs of colic in which the animal becomes restless, moves about aimlessly, respiratory rate goes up. There may be grinding of teeth. Later, the animal becomes recumbent and there is paddling of feet.

Causes

Sudden change in feed; overeating, etc.

Treatment

1. *Spasmovet* (Vetoquinol product): It contains Diclomine hydrochloride as injection./ *Dose:* 1 ml/20 kg BW by intramuscular route only.
   Cows, etc. 10–15 ml.
   Dog: 0.5 to 2 ml.
2. *Epidosin (TTK Pharma):* It is a very good smooth muscle relaxant (Valethamate bromide and Chlorbutol) and cervical dilator (during delivery), good for abdominal, urogenital colic and prolapse.
   Dose: Cows, etc. 10 ml/IM injection; dogs and cats 2.5 to 5 ml.
3. *SPAS (G. Glucotos and Co, Mumbai):* Inject 1 ml/25 kg BW.; cattle, horse 10–15 ml; sheep, goat 1–2 ml; dog 0.5–1 ml by intramuscular injection.

■ THELAZIOSIS (EYE WORM DISEASE)

Etiology

Thelazia species of worms.

These are minute threadlike worms found in the mucous membrane of conjunctiva. Larvae come out on the surface of the eye. These larvae are eaten by flies of Musca sp. These flies transmit infection into the eyes of other cattle, buffaloes, sheep and goats. The problem is more common in rainy season.

Diagnosis

1. Presence of Thelazia worms in conjunctiva.
2. Microscopic examination of tears will show eggs or larvae.
3. Flies storming around the eyes of animals.

Treatment

1. Ivermectin injection—0.2 mg per kg BW or 1 ml per 50 kg BW may be injected and if necessary, repeated after 15 days.
2. Levamisol: 5 mg/kg BW by SC Injection which may be repeated after 2 weeks. (Lemasol injection 30 ml vial, Zoetis product)

■ YOKE GALL

Yoke gall is an acute or chronic swelling of skin and SC tissue in working bullocks where yoke shaft rests (upper part of neck).

Treatment

In initial inflammatory stage, anti-inflammatory ointments may be applied such as Mastilep of Natural Remedies. Topicure of Natural Remedies may be applied.

If complicated with pus or necrosis, surgical incision and draining out of exudates is necessary.

1. *Homoeopathic drugs:* Give Hepar Sulph 200 1/2 teaspoonful and Silicia 200 1/2 teaspoonful once in 2–3 days. Silicia is helpful in dissolving fibrous tissue.
2. Give Calendula 30 (1/4 teaspoonful) twice daily and apply Calendula ointment for fast healing.
3. Calcaria florica 30, 1/2 teaspoonful, twice a day in chronic stage.
4. Safroid spray (100 ml) of Kepler once or twice a day.
5. *Avil injection:* In early acute stage, daily till swelling subsides.
6. Wisprec spray (Natural Remedies) twice a day.
7. *Exoheal (Intas):* Very good for yoke and rope galls, FMD, foot rot, dermatomycosis, mange, ringworm, etc.

■ NAVAL ILL IN CALVES

The umbilical cord at the time of birth may become infected due to unhygienic cutting of the cord and daily nonapplication of tincture of iodine or antiseptic ointments. Pus producing Staphylococci, streptococci, *E. coli*, Sph, necrophorous, etc. easily multiply in blood filled umbilicus.

Signs

The cut end of umbilicus becomes swollen and inflamed. There is fever, loss of appetite. Septicaemia may develop with spread of infection into the joints or joint ill. Later, pus forms in the umbilicus.

Treatment

1. Drain out the pus if it is found in umbilicus.

2. Immediately give homoeopathic drug Hepar Sulph 200 1/2 teaspoonful, and about 30 minutes later give Silicia 200, 1/2 teaspoonful, once in a day. Repeat them if necessary.

3. Inject antibiotics like Dicrysticine, Terramycin long-acting or Terramycin, long-acting (Zoetis), Enromycin (Byrocin 1 shot) or Seftifur gm (Merial). These injections should be able to treat the disease.

4. Colostrum must be fed as soon after birth (warm) as possible to prevent infection by internal immunity.

FILARIAL DERMATITIS IN CATTLE

Etiology: Filarial worms *Parafilaria multipapillosa* and *Parafilaria bovicola*. These worms enter into the skin by biting of flies (blood sucking). These flies also transmit the larvae of parasite into other cattle.

Signs: Mostly, the disease occurs in hot and humid season which is favourable for multiplication of flies. There are small elevated nodules on the skin with some redness around them. Later, these papules burst open and discharge some blood. Such lesions are mostly found on the neck, shoulders and around the eyes. Microscopically filarial worms or larvae can be found in the exudates. The discharge of blood from nodules takes 5 to 8 months for maturation of larvae into adult. The adult come out of skin.

Treatment: Treatment may not be required but if very severe, treatment may be given. Ivermectin injection 0.2 mg per kg BW SC may be given.

DISEASES OF EYES

It is not possible to deal with all the diseases of eyes in this manual but common conditions are given below:

Conjunctivitis: It may be acute with redness or purulent with pus-like exudates. I treat such cases by giving homoeopathic Argentum nitricum 1000 liquid given orally (Homoeopathic). It may be given in drop doses in small animals, 1/4 teaspoonful in calves, sheep and goats and 1 teaspoonful in large animals by mouth, mixed with a little water, once a day till recovery.

Other antibiotic eyedrops for eyes are:
a. *Gennol eyedrops of gentamycin* (Coles, Zenlab product).
b. *Flurr eyedrops.*
c. *Tobramycin eyedrops* (ICIN drops manufactured by Albes Healthcare Ltd, HP).
d. *Ciplox*, ciprofloxacian eyedrops (Cipla)—10 ml.
e. *Ciprocan D eyedrops* —15 ml with dexamethasone for allergic conjunctivitis.
f. *Otipet eyedrops* —contains gentamycin.
g. *Clotrimazole* (antifungal) betamethasone (antiallergic) and lignocaine (anti-inflammatory).

BAD ODOUR IN DOGS (SKIN)

Some dogs may emit bad body odour. This is usually due to secondary fungal infections of skin. First, bathe the dog with shampoo. When dry, dust Frecia (Derm care) powder over affected parts of the body twice daily. Dissolve *Luspur (100 ml) liquid (Kepler) in some water and apply liberally all over the body, allow to stand for 10–15 minutes* then wash off. *Sheen-n-Kleen shampoo (Venkys)* contains ketoconazole and removes dandruff and fungi. Apply on wet coat. Leave for 7–10 minutes and wash.

■ EAR INFECTIONS

Ear infections may be due to bacterial, fungal (yeast) or mites infection. The symptoms may be just itching in ears causing scratching by claws (pedal reflex) or there may be puslike discharge from ears.

Treatment

1. *Zotek-P eardrops* (Biomedica Remedies). It contains gentamicin (antibacterial), clotrimazole (antifungal), betamethasone (antiallergic) and lignocaine (anti-inflammatory).
2. *Otipet eardrops*: Otipet has similar contents as in Zotek.
   Use: Put 8 to 10 drops per ear once or twice a day. If there is no response, then antimite *injections of Ivermectin* may be given. Alternatively, *'Derm Care' soap* (of Zydus) may be used as shampoo to work up rich lather. The lather is allowed to work for 5 minutes and then washed off with clean water (caution: do not use in pups below 3 months and in nursing bitches).
3. *Otriel eardrops (Zydus AH, a division of Cadilla Healthcare):* Otriel eardrops contain clotrimazole (antifungal), ofloxacin (antibacterial), betamethasone (antiallergic), lignocaine HCL (pain killer).
   Presentation: 15 ml dropping bottle.
   Dose: 8 to 10 drops per ear, 2 or 3 time a day.
4. *Calm Eardrops (Scientific Remedies)*: Contains ofloxacin, beclomethasone, clotrimazole, and lignocaine like Zotek-P. Put 7–8 drops in each ear 2–3 times daily.

■ DRY EYES

Dry eyes, particularly in summer or dusty season may result in 'pedal reflex'. In such cases, use the following medicines for flushing by 'fresh tears'.

Zens Fresh Tears (product of Zenlabs Ethica Ltd, Goregaon, Mumbai). Use 3 times a day.

■ NAILS OF PETS

Nails of dogs may be trimmed (but never of cats) but not before the age of 3 months—special nail trimmers are available online or from pet shops. Care should be taken not to trim too much otherwise bleeding may occur. There is no fixed schedule for trimming. Only when nails produce discomfort to owners then trimming is done.

Nails are very important for confidence in cats hence nails should not be trimmed. Cats feel depressed by nail cutting.

■ OBESITY IN DOGS

Obesity may occur due to:
1. Overfeeding, particularly meat and eggs (yolk).
2. Hypothyroidism.
3. Insulinoma (tumour).
4. Feeding several times a day like human beings.

Hormonal cause can be diagnosed by laboratory tests of blood. To monitor, weigh the dog weekly at the same time of the day and on the same scale.

Complete change of food is better than modifying the food being used. Give more moist food to increase the volume and not the calories. Increase the exercise of the dog through walking or playing. Reduce the caloric contents of food but gradually and not suddenly. Provide raw vegetables like tomato if possible. Provide 30 to 50% calories through highly digestible cooked grain (starch). Provide dietary fiber such as bran (about 1 teaspoonful/day).

Fat may form 15 to 30% of diet. Omega 3 (n-3) fatty acids may be provided.

Overweight dogs result in complications such as arthritis, decreased immunity resulting in repeated infetions, heart and circulatory problems.

Homoeopathic Medicines

Phytolacca preparations: Commercial, e.g. Maxislim 5 drops in some water, daily.

ONION AND GARLIC TOXICITY IN PETS

Onions and garlic may be occasionally fed to pets as table scraps or mixed in pet food under mistaken belief of being good for health.

These vegetables produce haemolytic (destruction of RBCs) anaemia. The main toxic material is sodium propylthiosulphate which also causes methaemoglobin formation. N propyl disulphide also is a toxic factor. Even cattle, horses, sheep, goats besides dogs and cats may suffer from toxicity. Farmers may feed onions due to low market price.

Toxic dose in dogs is 30 g/kg BW of onions.

Symptoms

Lethargy, weakness, abdominal pain, vomiting, diarrhoea, tachycardia, dyspnoea, splenomegaly and anaemia within 24 hours after intake.

Treatment

Stop the onions or garlic as early as possible.

Give treatment for anaemia by injections of 'Dextran' as per manufacturers' instructions.

Sharkoferol syrup, given orally, 1 teaspoonful twice daily; 2–3 ml/kg BW daily till recovery. Repeat every 4–6 hours.

For diarrhea and vomitting: KOL suspension of Carus Lab Pvt Ltd.

Old Dogs' Support

1. *Synopet* (by Nuvo division of Intas)
   Indications:
   a. Joint supplement for supporting old dogs movement by protecting joint cartilage, ligaments, and tendons.
   b. Convalescence after operation.
   c. Remove stress.
   d. Dysplasia, arthritis, etc.
   Dose: Dogs up to 10 kg 4 g daily.
         10–20 kg 6 g.
         Above 20 kg 8 g.
         Cats up to 5 kg 2 g daily.
         Above 5 kg 4 g.

2. *Melonex suspension* (Nuvo/Intas) may be given on 1st day and (0.2 mg/kg) and 0.1 mg/kg BW daily, orally.
3. *Nerveon (Vetina)*: Contains methyl cobalamin, lycopene, selenium, B_1, B_6, etc.
   Indications: Repair of nerves, protects from free radicals.
   Dose: 1/2 to 2 tablets orally in food daily.
   Packing: 30 tablets.

▓ DIGESTIVE UPSETS IN DOGS AND CATS

1. *Zymopet (Nuvo division of Intas)*: All digestive enzymes in 30 ml bottle.
   Dose: Pups 0.5 to 1 ml BID.
           Small dogs 1 to 1.5 ml BID.
           Large dogs 1.5 to 2 ml BID.
           Cats 0.5 to 1 ml BID.
2. *KOL (Carus Lab):* Activated charcoal suspension
   Dose: 2–3 ml/kg BW every 12 hours or 1 bolus/10–15 kg BW. Repeat dose after 12 hours.
3. *Vetri Liv Pets (Venkys):* Appetiser, liver tonic.
   Dose: 5–10 ml twice daily.

▓ ATOPIC DERMATITIS IN DOGS

1. *Takapet* (Nuvo of Intas): Contains lipid based Tacrolimus and Alphatocopherol.
   Use: Spray on affected skin from 50 ml spray bottle.
2. *Dermachlor spray*: After bathing, spray from 15 cm distance on skin (not eyes and nose) and then dry the skin.

▓ ECTOPARASITES CONTROL

1. *Kiltix Collar* (Bayer product): It is a unique and very convenient collar (belt) which is to be stretched 2 to 3 times before use. Place the collar around dog's neck. Cut off the extra length of collar.
   a. Rapid action of Propoxur and Flumethrin in the collar is released from collar as fine powder which migrates along dog's coat and kills ticks starting from 24 hours after application.
   b. It works even if the dog gets wet in rain.
   c. Complete protection against ticks and fleas.
   d. Good tolerance towards killer ingredients.
2. *Butox powder* (MSD product): Remember that only 5% ticks are found in cattle body and 95% in sheds, tree bark, cracks, crevices, etc.
   Content: Deltamethrin
   Use: All animal species as spray or dip
           Ticks 2 ml per litre
           Mites 4 ml per litre
           Lice 1 ml per litre
           Flea 2 ml per litre
   Packing: 5, 15, 20, 50, 250 ml and 1 litre.
   For milk use: 0 day withdrawal.
   Meat: 20 days withdrawal time.

3. *Taktic liquid 12.5% EC (Amitraz 125 mg/ml; MSD product):* Mix 12.5% Taktic per litre of water for dropping on midline of the back of pigs, sheep and goats—4 ml for ticks.
   Cattle, buffaloes, camel: 4 ml for mites.
   Withdrawal period: 1 day for cows and buffaloes.
   For all small animals: 7 days.
   Packing: 15, 50, and 250 ml.
4. *Parid Pour On (Vets Farma):* For almost all ectoparasites. Each ml contains ivermectin 0.5% + benzyl alcohol.
   Pour on at midline of spine at the rate of 1 ml per 10 kg BW.
5. *Allgone (Hester product):* Contains Amitraz 125 mg/ml. Use as "Tactic" given above.
6. *Tik-Out (Alembic product):* Contains Cyper methrin. It is effective for 50 days after single application. It is fast oil-based insecticide against all ectoparasite.
   Use: Dissolve 1 ml Tik Out in 1 litre water and spray on body of the animal.
   For shed: Dissolve 20 ml Tik Out per litre and spray in shed (cracks, crevices, bark of trees).
   Packing: 30, 50, and 100 ml.

CANINE PELLAGRA

It is a kind of stomatitis mainly affecting tongue bluish inflamed with ulcerations in mouth and drooling of saliva and loss of appetite. In human beings, pellagra is mainly due to niacin deficiency but it can be said that the source of vitamin B being almost the same, it is generally multivitamin B deficiency disease.
   Treatment: *Beejet injection* (B_1, B_2, B_3, B_5, B_6, and B_{12} Vets Pharma).
   Give IM or IV 3 to 5 ml injection for 3 to 5 days or for 10 days on alternate days.

Glossitis or Sore Mouth

1. For this homoeopathic nitric acid 1000 liquid 5 ml may be purchased. Give 2–3 drops 3 times a day in a little water.
2. Boric acid 30 (homoeopathic liquid 5 ml): Give 1 drop morning evening in sugar pills.
3. Use Hexidine mouth wash or Betadine wash if Hexidine fails. Syringe may be used or a cotton swab on wooden stick.
4. If sore mouth due to vitamin deficiencies is seen, give B complex (Becosule) or Becom L daily for several days.

CONSTIPATION

Constipation may be due to diet less in fibre such as white bread, eggs, etc. Train the dog to go for regular walks to make the motion habitual. Give plenty of water all the time.

Homoeopathic drugs are excellent:

1. Opium 200 liquid (5 ml): Give 3–4 drops in mouth in morning.
2. Bryonia 200: Same way as opium.
3. Let the dog run after a ball which stimulates adrenalin and bowel movement. If it becomes problematic, give Dulcoflex or Dulcolax 1/2 or 1 tablet at night before sleep (in jiggery or honey).

Or give Esuphgoal husk: 1/2 to 1 teaspoonful in milk at night.

If no response, then enema may be given (50–100 ml olive oil or warm water or saline enema).

DEWORMING OF PETS

It is advised to do deworming of dogs every month starting from 1 month of age.

Examples of drugs used for deworming:

1. *Worm Trap (Petcare product):* Box of 10 tablets. Contains praziquantel, Pyrentel Pamoate and Febantel (Cargil marketing).
   Action: Acts against roundworms, hookworms (blood sucking), tapeworms and whipworms.
   Dose: 1 tablet per 10 kg BW orally in food or chocolate cover.

2. *Slayworm* (Merial product)—for dogs only. Contains above medicines in tablet form (Boxofio).
   Dose: 1 tablet per 10 kg BW.
   Control intermediate hosts such as fleas, mice and rats. Store in a cool dry place (marketed by Sanofi-Synthelabo India Pvt Ltd).

3. *Kiwof Puppy*—puppy dewormer. Oral suspension; contents are same as in the above 2 medicines. (SAVA VET PROD).
   Dose: 1 ml per kg BW, by dropper. (Save Healthcare Ltd; 507-B to 512, G.I.D.C. Estate Wadhwan City 363035, Surendranagar, Gujarat).

4. *Petantel Puppy (Pet Bovine Product):* Contains Pyrental Pamoate and Febantel as suspension. May be given to pups and kittens.
   Dogs: Dose 1 ml/kg BW.
   Cats: 1–3 ml per 3 kg BW.
   Do deworming at 2, 4, 6, 8, 10, and 12 weeks of age then monthly after 12 weeks.

5. *Drontal Plus (Bayer):* 1 tablet/10 kg BW × 3 days; Drontal Puppy: 1 ml per kg BW.

6. *Worm Tek*: Contains Pyrantel Embonate and Febantel active against hookworms, roundworms, tapeworms and whipworms, Ascarids, Toxocara, Taxascaris and Uncinaria.
   Dose: Give directly by mouth, 1 ml per kg BW. Use within 12 weeks after opening the bottle.

7. *Canworm (Vetina)*: Treats roundworms, tapeworms, hookworms, whipworms, giardia.
   Dose: Large dogs: 1 ml/kg BW.
   Puppies: 0.5 ml per kg BW.
   Packing: 30 ml.

HEAT STROKE OR HYPERPYREXIA (DOGS)

1. Give *Paracetamol* 1 tablet (1/2 in puppies) 4 hourly.
2. *Cold sponging of body.*
3. Adding a little *alcohol to water* helps dissipate heat.
4. *Ice water enema.*
5. *50% dextrose saline infusion*, 500–1000 ml daily to bring dehydration to normal. **Avoid over-infusion** otherwise pulmonary oedema may occur.
6. *Shift patient to AC room, if possible.*

Homoeopathic: Give 5–10 drops Glonoine 6 or 30 every 15–30 minutes till temperature returns to normal (very specific). Give plenty of vitamin C (500 mg) as chewable tablets (Limcee) 2–3 times a day.

■ IRRITABILITY IN DOGS
Causes

1. Separation and social anxiety.
2. Travelling stress.
3. Motion sickness.
4. Fireworks at Diwali.
5. Aggressiveness.
6. Destructive manners.

Trzatnient: 'Mind Calming Tablets' (VETINA product).

Contents: Chamomilla—45 mg.

Extract of ginger—45 mg.

Valerian root—45 mg per tablet.

Packing: 30 tablets of Mind Calming (Vetina, Pune).

Dose: Up to 5 kg: 1 tablet daily.

10–15 kg: 3 tablets daily.

Over 20 kg: 4 tablets daily.

Homoeopathic: Ignatia 200: 1–2 drops in sugar pills once/twice.

Staphysagria 1000: 2–3 drops in sugar pills/water twice a day.

Sepia 200: 2–3 drops twice a day as above.

■ CYANIDE POISONING

Hydrocyanic acid poisoning is common in ruminants. Hungry animals suddenly allowed to eat lush green plant growth or plants growing in soil with high nitrogen contents in soil or low phosphorus; wilted and young plants high in alkalinity in rumen increase the tate of absorption of HCN.

Signs: Animals rarely survive for more than 1 or 2 hours. Signs begin within 10 to 15 minutes after eating toxic plants. Signs are dyspnoea, anxiety, tremors, moaning and recumbancy. All symptoms are due to stoppage of oxygen exchange. Main effect is due to anoxia of brain from heart failure.

Treatment

1. Inject sodium nitrite 10–30 ml of 30% solution IV over 2 to 4 minutes.
2. Or inject 5 g sodium nitrite, 15 g sodium thiosulphate in 200 ml water for cattle and 1 g sodium nitrite and 3 g sodium thiosulphate in 50 ml water for sheep. Sometimes, much higher dose of 660 mg/kg BW combined with sodium nitrite 22 mg/kg BW gives good results.
3. Inject 1000 mg vitamin B_{12} per 60 kg BW.
4. Sodium thiosulphate heavy (above dose).
   Combined with cobaltous chloride (10.6 mg/kg BW).

Precautions

Be careful about avoiding overfeeding with sorghum species of grasses ('jwar', 'bajra', etc. specially if wilted).

■ HALITOSIS (FOUL SMELL FROM BREATH/SKIN)

This is observed in dogs due to poor oral hygiene or due to chronic digestive disorders, kidney diseases, liver diseases or due to nasal infections or pyorrhoea.

Treatment

1. Wash the mouth with equal parts of 3% hydrogen peroxide and water 2–3 times a day.
2. Dentastix (of Virbac) or Veggie (product of Virbac) available in 3 sizes may be used in small, medium or large dogs for cleaning of the mouth.
3. Dentopet paste: 70 g (Ektek Pharma) for cleaning/brushing mouth.
4. Dentopet spray for spray or povidone iodine spray (Tineta).
5. Hexidine or Betadine mouthwash.
6. Capsule Terramycin 250 mg 1 × 3 for 5 days.
7. Remove tartar from teeth.

■ LAMENESS

Hosts: Cattle, camel, sheep, goats, and horses.

Symptoms

Main sign is lameness due to osteitis, arthritis, or myositis or laminitis or pain and inflammation due to trauma or it may be due to pyrexia associated with viral or bacterial diseases. These drugs remove pain as well as fever.

Treatment

1. *Gluck*: Injection IM, IV or SC.
   Presentation: 15 ml vial (Bayer product): Main drug is Ketoprophen 100 mg/ml.
   Dose: Inject 1 ml per 33 kg BW for 3–5 days. In horses 1 ml per 45 kg BW, IV for 3–5 days.
2. Melonex injection containing meloxicam of several companies (Intas, Vets Pharma, Mankind, Intas Pet) can also be used.
3. *Inflavet injection* (Virbac): Meloxicam and paracetamol and lignocaine, 50 ml vial.
   Dose: 2–3 ml/33 kg BW, IM, IV, SC, injection.
4. Carpofen injection (Zydus): Single dose active for 3 days.
   Indications: Lameness, trauma, surgery dystocia, etc.
   Dose: Cattle, etc. 1–4 mg (2.4 ml) per kg BW, IM, IV, SC injection.
        Horse: 0.7 mg/kg BW.

Homoeopathic

Arnica 200 in some water may be given at the dose rate of 4–5 drops three times a day in small animals or about 1 ml in large animals.

■ CONVULSIONS

Convulsions means spasms in the body muscles, mostly in pets due to large variety of causes including genetic, parasitic, negative energy balance, protozoan diseases, poisonings, etc. Cause cannot be easily detected. Anticonvulsion drugs include phenobarbitol (Gardenal), diazepam (Calmpose, Valium), Carbamazepine (Mazetol, Tegretol, and phenytoin, Eptoin and Epsolin) in tablets or injections.
   Calmpose 2 ml injection/10 mg; dose: 0.5 to 1 mg per kg BW.

Chronic Locomotor Disease in Dogs

Sometimes dogs may suffer from limpindg or lameness due to unknown causes. To remove this symptom and for slow self cure following treatment can be attempted besides steps given under the topic of lameness.

1. *Tolfine* (Vetoquinol): Contains tolfenamic acid as injection.
   Dose: Dog 4 mg per kg BW (1 ml for 10 kg BW).
   IM once daily. It may be repeated if needed after 24 hours.
2. *Neurobion injections:* 0.5–2 ml, IM × 7 (in 14 days).
3. *Arnica 200 (Homoeopathic medicine):* 1 drop or 10–12 globules twice a day or if it fails give Arnica 1000 (1M) in same dose.

Febrile Syndrome in Cats

Chronic recurrent fever of unknown causes:

1. *Dose:* Same as in dogs.
2. *Natrum mur 1000:* 1–2 drops in water once or twice a day. This is wonderful drug for chronic fever of any origin.

Chapter 23

Cancer Treatment

There are only a few types of cancers which may be successfully treated by chemotherapy. They are mentioned below.

Canine and Feline Leukemia

Cause: Feline leukemia virus (FeLV).

Clinical Picture

1. Enlargement of lymph nodes—splenomegaly.
2. Tumóurs palpable in abdomen.
3. Anaemia
4. Intermittent pyrexia.
5. Sickness without age dependence.
6. Vertical and horizontal (from mother) transmission.
7. Sick cats can survive for years with disease.
8. Virus destroys T lymphocytes hence immunodeficiency.

Treatment

Vinecristine injection (Cipla and Biochem products)

In dogs 0.3 ml per 10 kg BW strictly IV injection in normal saline. No other medication may be given. Repeat weekly 3 times.

Prednisone: 2 mg/kg/day PO (peroral/for 1st week; 1.5 mg/kg/ PO for 7 days then 0.5 mg/kg/PO for 7 days).

▣ WARTS (PAPILLOMA)

Canine Oral Papilloma

Electrocauterisation may be tried on limited scale.

Cutaneous Warts

In all animals particularly common in cattle.

Pure carbolic acid: Apply with glass rod or pure trichloracetic acid may be painted on warts.

Or Externally apply the following mixture:
   Salicylic acid 2.5 g.
   Lactic acid 2.5 g.
   Flexible collodion 15 g.

Or

Alcohol 120 ml.
Salicylic acid 3.5 g.
Paint daily for 7 to 10 days.

Homoeopathic

Give Thuza 1000: 1 teaspoonful daily by mouth in some water.
Wartex liquid (Q) apply externally daily.
Carcinocin Q: 5 drops 3 times a day for carcinomas.

Squamous Cell Carcinoma (Horn Cancer, Cancer of Eye, Ear; Cancer of Sheep)

I have treated about 70% cases of horn cancer by the following steps:
1. Remove as much cancer tissue as possible surgically (use 'Jack shot' injection to stop bleeding).
2. I prepared protein antigen by ultracentrifugation of cancer tissue homogenate.
3. Inject the protein antigen SC on neck and around the skin just around the affected horn.
4. Inject BCG vaccine around the affected horn (about 0.25 mL per point).
5. Do dressing of horn daily after dehorning (refer Australian Vet Journal 56, 1980, 509-510).

Chapter 24

Sure Shots of Homoeopathy*

I cannot write about all the good medicines of homoeopathy in this small handbook but I am mentioning some 'sure shots' of my 40 years in practice.

1. *The mixture of 9 biochemic medicines (Cholera mixture)* given under chapter of diarrhoea in calves works like magic to stop diarrhoea—even shooting diarrhoea—if given in some hot water at 15 to 30 minutes intervals by mouth—dose 1/2 to 1 easpoonful.

   I also give Croton 6 mixed in 1–2 drops in sugar pills or even clean water in between the above mixture.

2. *Hepar Sulf*: Hepar Sulf 200 is a wonderful medicine which will cure any disease with pus formaton, particularly in skin, mammary glands, etc.

   I treated cases of 'crops of abscesses' in several people when allopathic medicines failed to cure permanently.

   In chronic cases, removal of pus or pus-like exudates, e.g. from udder. I give Hepar Sulf 200 1 teaspoonful 3 times a day and Silicia 200 also 1 teaspoonful, twice a day.

3. For acute inflammation with redness and swelling, *Belladonna 1000* 2–3 drops in 2–3 hours usually stops the problem such as throat infection. This I follow with Mecuric cor 200 2–3 drops to remove infection.

   Aconite 30 4–6 globules may be given every 20 minutes or so to help Belladonna. This is one of the best treatments of fever.

4. If there is puslike exudates in the eyes of any species of animal or man, 2–3 drops of Argentum nitricum 1000 given morning and evening by mouth will cure the infection.

5. *Nitric Acid 1000:* If there is any ulcer in mouth or tongue 1 or 2 drops of nitric acid will cure the ulcer in 12 hours. If not, repeat 12 hourly (best in human beings)

6. *Acidity and gastric or duodenal ulcers:*

   I have cured with a few exceptions cases of severe acidity and gastric ulcers by giving the following medicines:

   a. Argentum nitricum 1000: 2 drops once or twice a day on empty stomach

   b. Hydrochloric acid 30: 7–8 globules twice a day.

   c. Sooktyn (Alarsin) ayurvedic tablets: 2 after breakfast 2 after lunch and 2 after dinner. This may be continued for a month or so along with increase in intervals of dosing and reduction of tablets gradually.

7. *Bad mothering instinct (not allowing milk feeding to newborn calf):* This is sometimes observed in cows of exotic breeds or mares. In such cases, give 1/2 teaspoonful of Silicia 200 in some water by mouth. If necessary, repeat in the evening.

---

* *Note:* Use these homoeopathic medicines in consultation with a qualified homoeopath only.

8. *Deformed bones anywhere in the body:* Particularly in calves or heifers deformed legs with hooklike curvature of hoof and fetlock is common. In such cases, I have cured after several weeks of giving Hekla Lava 200 once a day to affected animal. Calcaria florica 30: 2 drops may also be given twice a day.

   I have used these medicines to treat cervical spondylosis or frozen shoulder of self but in small (2 drops of Hekla lava 200 and 1 drop of calcaria florica once or twice a day). This may also be accompanied by mild shoulder exercise (rotational).

9. *Ferrum phos*: Ferrum phos 1000 is an extraordinary medicine which has treated without fail cases of filariasis (hydrocoele, elephantiasis, or filarial swellings anywhere in the body) by giving 2–3 drops by mouth, if necessary for a few more days resulting in a smiling patient because there is no cure for filariasis in man in alopathy.

10. *Iridocyclitis*: I have treated permanently my own problem of iridocyditis (inflammation of iris) by taking Ferrum phos 1000 in 2–3 days and Ferrum phos 12 × tablets (3–4) twice a day for several days. There is no reliable therapy for this in allopathy. Belladonna 1000 may be taken as few drop doses once in a week.

11. *Glonoine: Glonoine 1000* given in 2–3 drop doses to patients of migraine (hemicrania) have been cured permanently. This dose given in clean or tasteless mouth may be repeated at 2–3 days intervals till the attacks stop.

    It is better ot minimise or stop eating of cheese, meat, raw onions as far as possible.

12. *Enlarged prostate*: Enlarged prostate is a big problem of almost all old persons. More the age more are the chances. The main attention should be given to the symptom of:

    a. Post-urination dribbling of urine.

    b. Frequent urge for urination (1, 2 or 3 hours).

    c. Faeces comes out as a ribbon.

    d. Burning of urethra, occasionally.

    The best diagnosis is by ultrasonography which shows the size of prostrate and retention of urine. Treat as early as possible.

    Medicines:

    a. *Sabal serrulata 30*: 7–8 globules should be taken 3–4 times a day

    b. *Staphysagria 30*: 7–8 globules morning and evening

    c. 'Prostina' capsules (Ayurvedic) of Dey Pharma, Kolkata

    d. 'Prostone' 50 of J.V.S. Pharmaceutical Co, 10–20 drops of this homoeopathic medicine may be given 3 times a day.

    Much more can be written about homoeopathic medicines but I do not want to defeat the purpose of a manual by making the book too big.

13. *Calendula*: Calendula, a homoeopathic medicine is a wonderful drug which not only cures any kind of damaged soft tissue (wound) but also removes infection. This medicine can be taken as Calendula 6 or 30, 6–7 globules can be taken by mouth 2–4 times a day. Calendula ointment or Calendula spray can also be used for external use. I have been using this as ointment for treatment of dozens of cases of wound brought to our hospital.

14. *Phosphorus*: Phosphorus 200 liquid can be administered as liquid 1 to 3 drops given orally in some water to stop bleeding from anywhere.

a. blood in milk

b. bleeding in cases of ROP

c. vomiting due to gastritis or presence of blood with diarrhoea in dogs. In such cases, it should be repeated at 1/2 an hour interval if vomiting of blood or bloody diarrhoea is more severe.

15. *Ignatia*: Ignatia is the drug which removes depression and sadness after loss of pup in bitch or death of calf or youngone. For this, give Ignatia 200 in repeated doses till the mother feels cheerful. I use this drug in 1–2 drop doses whenever I feel lonely or somewhat depressed.

16. *Arsenicum album 1000*: This medicine given in 1 or 2 drop doses by mouth in poultry in cases of Gumboro disease (IBD) or even Newcastle disease gives results in 15–20 minutes. The bird with closed eyes and looking close to death opens the eyes. It should then be given plenty of dextrose and ORS mixture to drink. It may start moving about and will try to drink lot of water. The dose may be repeated 2–3 times a day which will save large percentage of poultry.

17. *Graphites:* Graphites can be given orally as 6 or 12 dilution in water or globules for 'cracks' anywhere in the body. It is most efficient to cure 'anal fissure', a kind of cut or tear in the anus particularly in human beings. Graphites 'Hadensa' or Hemmamelis cream will soon cure the most miserable condition of the disease. Nitric acid 1000 may also be given as 1 or 2 drops in 2–3 days. Sulphur 200 can also help like graphites and nitric acid.

18. *Ledum:* Ledum is a wonderful medicine for a localised pain in back (lumbago) or injury by a sharp object like nail, thorn, etc. whish is very painful due to nerve injury. Ledum 30 or 200 taken in water or globules works very well.

19. *Soriafit (Medisynth)* a homoeopathic proprietary drop combination given in 10 drops 3 times a day cured psoriasis (itching, scaliness of entire body) of about 20 years duration in a few weeks. It also relieves chronic inflammation.

20. *Dysentery*: Dysentery means passing out of loose stools along with mucous and blood. Dysentery may cause intestinal tenesmus (spasms). For this, Mercury corrosivus or Aloe in 200 potency given as 8–10 globules on clean mouth will soon stop amoebic or bacillary dysentery. 'Dyskoll' of Medisynth company also is a good medicine.

21. *Renal calculi or stones*: Berberis vulgaris Q given in drop doses (5 to 10) several times a day will help in flushing out of painful stones from ureter or bladder. 'Rinakoll', a combination of homoeopathic medicines which also contains Berberis Q, given in 5 ml (teaspoonful) dose every 2 hours in acute conditions in adult will relieve pain in urinary system (renal colic) and calculi, if any.

22. *Allergic cough:* I have cured almost invariably cough due to dust, pollens, etc. which is troublesome with sneezing in the morning by giving:

a. Bromium (or Bromine) 30, 10 to 12 globules 2–3 times a day.

b. *Blatta orientalis* 200—2 or 3 drops once everyday.

'Kofeez', a homoeopathic combination (Medisynth) given as 5–10 ml dose twice or thrice a day is claimed to cure whooping cough, a troublesome cough.

23. *Corallium 12 or 30:* If it is given and repeated every 10–30 minutes, it is extremely good for whooping cough which comes nonstop like gunshots in bouts.

24. *Cuprum met:* It is one of the best medicines for spasms in intestine lading to so severe pain like a dagger pushed into abdomen (localised). I cured my own case

on one occasion when I was thinking of going to medical college hospital in Ranchi. But cuprum 30 dissolved the localised pain within 15–20 minutes. Cuprum 30 and Zin 200 also relieve painful spasms of leg muscles or fidgety restless legs.

25. *Hekla Lava:* It is a wonderful drug having action on all kinds of bone abnormalities such as cervical spondylitis with pain in the neck and upper arm. In such cases, it is better to give Hekla Lava 200 daily once or twice as liquid drops or in sugar pills along with calcaria florica 30 which will remove skeletal overgrowth and pain associated with it due to pressure on nerves. I have cured abnormalities of leg bone by these medicines. Hekla Lava also cures periodontitis if given in early stage.

26. *Floric acid:* Floric acid also helps in treating cervical spondylitis when given for several weeks in 30 potency.

27. *Belladonna:* Belladonna 200 or 1000 taken in drop doses will stop acute inflammation anywhere in the body. I stop throat infection (soreness) by taking a few drops once or twice. It also relieves congestive headache.

28. *Bryonia 200:* It is also a good medicine to treat upper respiratory infections and also helps in removing constipation due to inactive rectal movement.

29. *Opium 200:* I myself take a few drops of this drug once only and get relieved from severe constipation.

30. *Rumex 200:* A few drops given sometime before sleep followed by a spoonful (after 20–30 minutes) of cough syrup like Corex, or Torex, etc. generally provides sound coughless sleep.

31. *Hypericum 200:* A few drops of this medicine which may have to be repeated early is good to relieve neuralgic pain such as over or around eyes or facial neuralgia.

    Apis mel 30: Taken in globules relieves oedema due to any cause particularly swelling due to bite of bees, wasps, etc.

32. Colocynth 30 or 200 dilution may be taken in globules or water to relieve colic (abdominal)particularly if patient feels relief by pressure, massage or hot foamentation. This may relieve colic in a short time.

    It is also one of the best medicines to relieve sciatica (slip disc, etc.) along with complete rest to vertebral column.

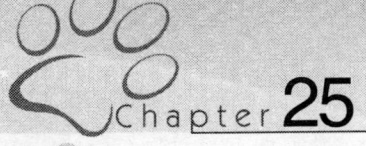

Chapter 25

Major Blood Diseases

◼ ANAEMIA

Anaemia means reduction in haemoblobin per unit volume of blood. There are several causes of anaemia which are more common in animals and including ruminants and pets.

Nutritional Anaemia

This is the commonest form of ill health and poor production in animals which is greatly ignored by most of the field doctors. I make it a point to take two steps as almost essential before taking case details.

1. Take temperature (rectal) of the animal and even bird.
2. Measure haemoglobin if the condition is moderate or poor.
3. See the colour of conjunctiva (to detect paleness/anaemia). In Australia, a coloured reference card is used to compare colour of conjunctiva which indicates gram of haemoglobin/dl. Impractical work of blood collection and laboratory work is avoided unless the problem is serious.

Common Nutritional Causes of Anaemia in Cattle

1. *Iron deficiency*: Mainly due to nonavailability of balanced nutritional formula, feeding of dry, poor quality straw, etc. Almost 75% of village cattle in states like MP, UP, Rajasthan, Bihar and probably also in Maharashtra and many other states are anaemic, unthrifty and unfit for farm work or milk yield or meat production in case of sheep and goats.
2. *Copper deficiency*: Copper in traces is also essential for synthesis of haemoglobin and sources being common, both are deficient.
3. *Zinc*: Zinc is not important for anaemia but its deficiency is also a part of the trio which results in poor skin health and skin diseases.
4. Cobalt deficiency.

Treatment

For list of drugs for anaemia see drug index.

1. Ferritas injections (Intas) 10 ml vial.
2. *Ferritas bolus:* 5 × 1 packet (Intas).
3. *Ferrimin Syrup:* Ekta Pharma.
4. Livoferol.
5. Sharkofenol (Alembic) syrup.
6. *Feriate iron sucrose injection:* 20 mg iron per ml (not for newborn or premature pups). Dilute with sterile normal saline to contain 0.5 to 2 mg iron per ml. Infuse in 15 minutes if given IV

7. *Fe-folate*: It is a syrup mainly for pets. Contains iron, folic acid and methyl cobalamin. Give 5 ml twice daily, particularly during pregnancy and lactation— 5 ml twice a day.

Anaemia due to Blood Loss: The biggest common cause of anaemia due to blood loss in animals are blood sucking worms, mainly Haemonchus species in sheep, goat and cattle and Bunostomum in cattle. Severe Oesophagostomum infection is so severe as to result in lack of iron and other minerals in ruminants. Regular deworming of sheep, goats and cattle is a must to stop the chances of these most harmful parasites. Ivermectin is produced by almost all veterinary pharmaceutical companies and the best advantage of Ivermectin is that it is available in injectable form, avoiding requirement of attendents and secondly, it kills almost all endoparasites and skin parasites also. Some common Ivermectin preparations are listed below.

1. *Mectin (Alembic; Ivermectin 1%):* It kills all worms listed above and even heartworms of dogs, and also ticks, lice mange, etc. (WHO certified).
   Presentation: 10 ml and 20 ml for SC injection.
   Dose: 200 micrograms (0.2 mg) per kg BW (about 1 ml per small animal).
2. *Closal bolus*: 150 mg/ml suspension or 1 gm/bolus (Alembic). This kills larvae and adult stages of liver fluke, GI roundworms including Haemonchus sp and Bunostomum nasal bot (Oestrous ovis) of sheep and Melophagus of sheep.
   Dose: Ectoparasites: 1 ml/10 kg BW.
          Endoparasites: 1 ml/15 kg BW.
3. *Trumectin (Zydus)*: Ivermectin 10 mg/ml injection.
   Dose: Cattle, sheep, goats: 0.2 mg/kg BW.
         Dog: 0.05 —0.2 mg/kg BW by SC injection.

Anaemia due to blood loss such as due to cancer, uterine bleeding, fractures, wounds have to be treated as given under different topics. Treatment for anaemia may be continued; other rare causes are haematuria, etc.

Anaemia due to blood protozoa: This is one of the most common causes of anaemia and has to be diagnosed and treated first for haemoprotozoa and then for anaemia. Refer to the topic of blood protozoan diseases.

Megaloblastic anaemia: This is more common in human beings and sometimes in dogs but not in ruminants and horses.

Treatment

1. Folic acid 5 mg daily for 2 or more months
2. *Vitamin B$_{12}$*—100 mcg IM daily for 7 days and 7 injections on alternate days and 7 injections weekly.

Chronic kidney diseases can also cause anaemia, mainly in dogs because erythropoietin produced in kidney becomes deficient. Erythropoietin is essential for RBC development in bone marrow. The only way to treat anaemia in such cases is to treat or control kidney disease. Use Rubenal 300 (Vetoquinol) using 1/2 to 3 tablets twice a day to control chronic kidney function.

■ LEUKOPENIA

Brief summary of blood changes:

Neutropenia

Less number of neutrophils occurs as response to toxaemia or endotoxaemia or enhanced migration of neutrophils to tissues. 'Granulocytopenic disease of calves' which may be due to poisoning by furazolidone. Prolonged septic focus (pyometra, empyema, pneumonia) may also cause neutropenia.

Lymphopenia

Commonly occurs in early stages of acute viral diseases such as hog cholera, quine viral arteritis. Lymphopenia also occurs as a part of severe stress response or administration of glucocorticoids.

Eosinopenia

Occurs in response to glucocorticosteroid administration, severe stress (cold, heat, toxaemia) severe enteropathogenic infections like typhoid, salmonellosis.

Panleakocytopenia

It is common in braken fern poisoning, chronic sulphonamide toxicosis, chlorpromazine drugging, toluene, fungal toxins, chloramphenicol toxicity.

Treatment should be directed at removal of the cause. Leucopenia may reduce resistance to secondary infections.

■ LEUKOCYTOSIS

Lymphocytosis

Causes of lymphocytosis are generally due to chronic bacterial diseases like tuberculosis, brucellosis, fungal infections. Very high lymphocytosis occurs in lymphocytic leukemia.

Neutrophilia

Neutrophilia may be associated with pyogenic infections, pneumonia, mastitis, etc. Subacute or chronic bacterial diseases usually cause neutrophilia without increase in band neutron; hils (immature). Slight neutrophilia also occurs during recovery stage of anaemia. High neutrophilia also occurs in pyogenic infections (metritis, mastitis, pneumonia) and septicaemia.

Eosinophilia

Main causes are:
1. Parasitic infections (ecto or endo).
2. Intestinal lymphosarcoma in horses.
3. Allergic conditions (mainly pollens, etc.).
4. Exhaustion or deficiency of adrenal corticosteroids.
5. Eosinophilic myeloproliferative disease in horses.

Monocytosis

Monocytosis in general is indicative of chronic infections such as tuberculosis and fungal infections. Immunological diseases or after vaccinations.

Abnormal White Cell Function

Abnormal white cell function can be congenital due to Chediak Higashi syndrome or bovine leukocyte adhesive deficienty. It can also be due to iron deficiency, mycotoxins, starvation, etc.

▉ PLATELET DISORDERS

Clinically thrombocytopenia must be suspected if there are petechial or ecchymotic haemorrhages in the body. (mucosa, skin, nose, eyes, etc.). Bleeding time (BT) is also prolonged (normal—5 to 10 minutes); there is prolonged bleeding after blood collection. There may be bleeding from nose (epistaxis), bowels (melena). These signs together are called purpura occurs if platelet count falls below 500/ml.

Thrombocytopenia may be caused by:
1. Immune mediated diseases.
2. Increased destruction in severe trauma.
3. Drug induced, by drugs which depress bone marrow.
4. Virus infections like hog cholera/swine fever in which haemorrhages all over the body are characteristic:
    – Bovine virus diarrhoea
    – Theileriosis
    – Bovine leukaemia
    – Salmonellosis
    – Ehrlichia canis infection
    – Babesiosis
    – Septicaemia
    – Hepatopathy
    – Peritonitis
Disseminated intravascular coagulopathies (poor prognosis).

Treatment

1. Treatment can be directed only at the primary disease. Low molecular weight heparin can be injected to prevent hypercoagulable states.
2. *Styptic (Himalaya):* Can be used in moderate bleeding conditions such as epistaxis, blood in milk, gastrointestinal bleeding, uterine bleeding, traumatic bleeding, surgical bleeding, etc.
    Dosage: Cows, buffaloes, horses and camels: 1–2 boli, twice daily.
    Calves and foals: 1 bolus twice daily.
    Sheep and goats: 1/2 bolus twice daily.

▉ BLOOD PARAMETERS IN DOGS: NORMAL REFERENCE RANGE

Biochemical Values		Hematological Values		Blood Parameters: Alteration in Diseases Biochemical Changes	
Glucose mg/dl	60–125	Erythrocytes 106/μL	5.5–8.5	Liver disorders	ALT, ALP, Bilirubin
Cholesterol mg/dl	112–328	Hemoglobin g/dl	12–18	Pancreatitis	Amylase, lipase
Protein g/dl	5.5–7.5	PCV%	37–54	Hypoadre-nocorticoid	Cholesterol, ALP, GlucoseK, P

Contd...

Biochemical Values		Hematological Values		Blood Parameters: Alteration in Diseases Biochemical Changes	
Albumin g/dl	2.6–4.3	MCV fl	66–77	Hyper-thyroidism	Cholesterol
Globulin g/dl	2.3–4.5	MCH pg	19.9–24.5	Diabetes	Glucose
A-G ratio	0.75–1.9	MCHC%	32–36	Rickets	ALP, Ca/P
BUN mg/dl	7–27	Platelets 103/µL	200–500	Renal failure	BUN, creatinine, K, P, Ca
Creatinine mg/dl	0.4–1.8	TLC 103/µL	6000–17000	Infection	Protein, globulin, albumin, A-G ratio
ALT (SGPT) IU/L	5–60	DLC ↓		Ehrlichiosis	ALP, ALT, globulin, albumin, A-G rate
AST (SGOT) IU/L	5–55	Neutrophils%	60–77	Babesiosis	Bilirubin, ALT
Alk Phos (ALP) IU/L	10–150	Lymphocytes%	12–30	*Hematological changes*	
Amylase IU/L	500–1500	Monocytes%	3–10	Acute infection	TLC neutrophils, lymphocytes
Lipase IU/L	100–500	Eosinophils%	2–10	Chronic infection	TLC lymphocytes, neutrophils
Bilirubin mg/dl	0.1–0.6	Basophils%	0–1	Anemia	Erythrocytes, Hb, PCV
Calcium mg/dl	8.7–11.8			Allergy	Eosinophils, basophils
Phosphorus mg/dl	2.9–6.2			Ehrlichia	Lymphocytes, platelets
Sodium mEq/L	140–154				
Potassium mEq/L	3.8–5.6				

■ BLEEDING DISORDERS

Epistaxis: Bleeding from nose.

Hematemesis: Vomitting of blood.

Uterine bleeding: Metrorrhagia.
Traumatic bleeding.
Surgical bleeding.

Hemogalactia: Blood in milk.

Hematuria: Blood in urine.

Treatment

1. *Styptic (Himalaya) bolus:*
   Cows, etc. 1–2 boli twice daily.
   Calves and foals 1 bolus twice daily.
   Sheep and goats 1/2 bolus twice daily.
2. *Addchrome injection* (G. Loucotas Co)—0.33 mg per kg BW. Generally, 12 ml IM (deep).
3. *Zak shot injection (Carus Laboratories):* Inject as advised by manufacturer.

4. *Phosphorus 200*: Homoeopathic; give orally 1/2 teaspoonful in cows, etc. oral and 6–8 drops in small animals, dogs and cats; repeat hourly or 2 hourly.

Species	PCV %	Haemo- globin (g/dl)	Erythro- cytes (106/μL)	MCV (fl)	Leuko- cytes (x103/μL)	Neutro- phil %	Lympho- cyte %	Mono- cyte%	Eosin- ophil %	Bas- ophil
Cattle	24–46	8–15	5–10	40–60	4–12	15–45	47–75	2–7	2–20	0–2
Buffalo	30–40	11–13	6–8	40–55	6–7	28–30	60–65	7–8	2–9	0–1
Horse	32–48	10–18	6–12	34–58	6–12	32–75	25–60	1–8	1–10	0–3
Sheep	27–45	9–15	9–15	28–40	4–12	10–50	40–75	0–6	0–10	0–3
Goat	22–38	8–12	8–18	16–25	4–13	30–48	50–70	0–4	1–8	0–1
dog	37–55	12–18	5.5–8.5	60–77	6–17	60–70	12–30	3–10	2–10	Rare

■ HABIT BREAKING FORMULA

1. Bad habits of eating undesirable things (fecal matter):
   Tablets: Fecal Detergent (Vetina).
   Contents: Monosodium glutamate (MSG) 200 mg.
   Oleoresis capsicum 0.021 mg
2. *Chewable, chicken flavour tablets:*
   Dose: Dogs up to 5 kg 1 tablet daily.
   5–10 kg 2 tablets daily.
   10–15 kg 3 tablets daily.
   15–20 kg 4 tablets daily.
   Packing: 30 tablets.

■ PET IDENTITY CHIP

One implant provides ownership proof for lifetime.

Features: Safe with no side effects.
   Painless insertion process.
   Cannot be lost or changed.
   No geographical boundaries.
   15 digit number for electronic identification.
   Sizes: 2.12 × 12 mm
   1.5 × 9 mm

Sites of implant: Subcutaneous implant the transponder on dorsal midline just cranial (front) of scapula.
   Or subcutaneously in midway portion of neck.
   Packing: 1 × 10 units.
   (Both the above products: contact Vetina Distributors, Pune; e-mail: customerservice@vetina.com; customer care number: 020-26633615).

Chapter 26

Livestock General Information

ANIMAL POPULATION AND PRODUCTION

Animal industry has acquired vast development after independence particularly in the last three decades. There are 20.5 million workers involved in livestock farming and production (National Sample Survey, 66th survey). India has only 2.29% of total land of the world but it has 10.71% of world's livestock population.

India is the largest milk producer in the world with animal population, tabled below (volume 40, Pashudhan, January 2014).

Veterinary facilities hospital polyclinics—10,094.

Veterinary dispensaries—21, 269.

Veterinary aid and stockmen/mobile dispensaries—25, 555.

Value of output from livestock in Indian economy (GOI32014)—₹ 537537 crores (about 65% milk, 20% meat, 4% eggs, dung 7%, 1% silk and honey, others 3%).

Livestock Industrial Production

- 146.3 million tonnes of milk in 2014–2015 with 5% growth (largest milk producer of the world).
- Per capita milk availability—290 g (2011–2012); very low; yearly.
- Egg production —78.48 billion eggs in 2014–2015 with 5% growth.
- Estimated (2016–2017)—83.11 billion eggs.
- Per capita egg availability—55 eggs.
- Export of poultry products (2011–2012)—₹ 458 crores.
- Poultry meat production (2011–2012)—2.47 million tonnes.
- Growth of 13% was recorded in total meat production in 2011–2012—5.5 million tonnes.
- Wool production in 2011–2012 was 44.73 million kg; growth in wool was 4%.
- Meat production in 2014–15—6.7 million tonnes.
- Wool and hair production in 2014–15—48.1 million kg.

Farmers' income: Gujarat 24.4%; Haryana 24.2%; Punjab 20.2%; Bihar 18.7% (Planning Commission 2012).

Uses—Cattle, Buffalo and Goat Animals in Milk

Animals in milk mean the animal's who contribute towards production of milk. The total number of animals in milk in the country is 116.77 million numbers.

Fluctuation in Animal Population: 19th Livestock Census, 2012

- Total population (calf, buffalos, sheep, goat, pigs, horses, mules, donkeys, camels, yak, mithun 512.05 million (2012) decreased by 3.33% from previous census. Gone up in Gujarat (5.36%), UP (14.01%), Punjab (9.57%), Bihar (8.56%), Sikkim (7.96%), Meghalaya (7.41%), Chhattisgarh (4.34%).

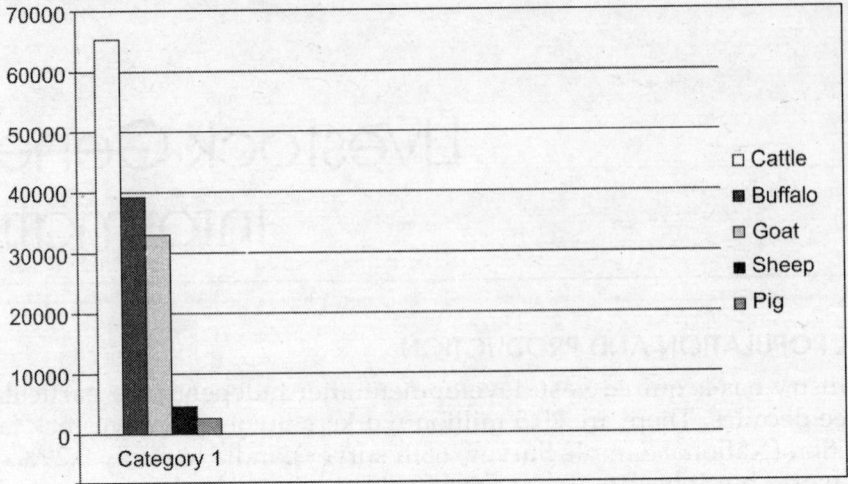

Fig. 26.1: Number of household enterprises having cattle, buffalo, sheep, goats and pigs (showing number of NH in "000)

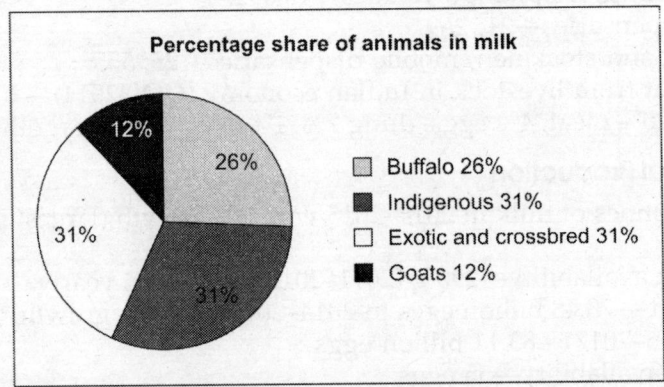

Fig. 26.2: Percentage share of animals in milk

- Milch cows and buffaloes has gone up from 111.69 to 118.59 millions.
- Cows and buffaloes have increased by 77.04 million to 80.52 million (4.51%).
- Cow population has gone up by 6.52%.
- Buffalo population has gone up by 7.99%.
- Exotic breeds have gone up by 4.95%.
- Sheep declined by 9.07% (from 2007).
- Goats declined by 3.82% (from 10.29 million).
- Pigs declined by 7.54%.
- Horses and ponies have increased by 2.08%.
- Mules have gone up by 43.34%.
- Camels have declined by 22.22%.
- Donkeys have declined by 27.22%.
- Poultry have increased by 12.39% to 792.2 millions, 2012.
- Mithun and yak have gone up 12.98% and 7.64% respectively.
- Dogs have declined from 19.08 million (2007) to 11.67 million (2012).
- Rabbits have increased from 0.424 million by 39.55% (possibly due to broiler rabbit farming).

- Elephants have gone up by 1000 to 22000.
- Buffalo milk is declined by 56% in rural areas.
- Female buffaloes have gone up to 10% in rural areas.

Sheep (% of India)

- Andhra Pradesh 40.57, Karnataka 14.73%.
- Rajasthan 13.95%, Tamil Nadu 7.36%.
- J and K 5.21%, Maharastra 3.97%.

Goats

Goats make 26.40% of the total Indian livestock which is 135.17 million goats (2012 census) highest number about 16% of Indian goats are reared in Rajasthan. About 29% are reared in UP, Bihar and West Bengal.

Indigenous cattle population has dropped by 65% during 2007 to 2012.

Poultry (Livestock Census 2012)

Poultry consists of generally three categories, namely, fowls, ducks, turkey, and others. The total poultry population in the country is 729.2 million numbers.

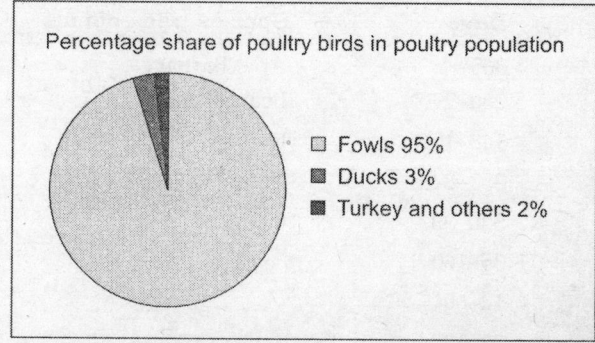

Fig. 26.3: Percentage share of poultry birds in poultry population

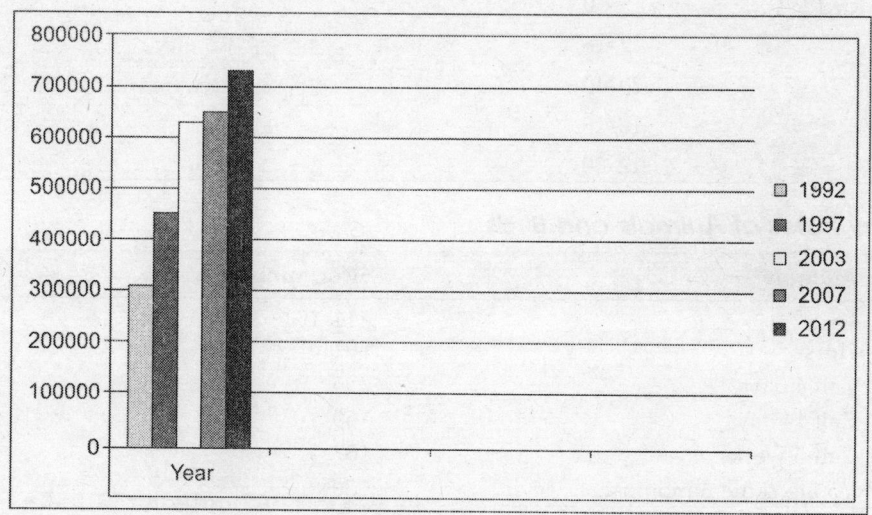

Fig. 26.4: Poultry Population during 1992–2012

Heart rates (Beats/minute)

Animal	Average	Range
Human	70	58–104
Ass	50	40–56
Camel	30	25–32
Cat	120	110–140
Cow	55	45–70
Dog	—	100–130
Elephant	35	22–53
Giraffe	66	—
Goat	90	70–135
Guinea pig	280	260–400
Horse	44	23–70
Lion	40	—

Gestation period in animals

Species livestock	Days	Species wild animals	Days
Ass	365	Ape, Barbary	210
Cattle	280–290	Bear, Black	214
Goat	148–156	Bison	275
Horse, heavy	333–345	Camel	410
Horse, light	330–337	Coyote	60–64
Mink	35–160		
Silver fox	12–60		
Coypou (nutria)	32–120		
Rhesus monkey	15–30		
Domestic fowl	15–30		
Turkey	12–16		
Pigeon	20–40		
Duck	16–28		
Goose	12–30		

Respiratory Rates of Animals and Birds

Animals	Per minutes
Foal	14–15
Horse	9–10
Calf 4 days	56
Calf 14 days	50
Calf 5 weeks	37
Young cattle 6 months	30

Contd...

Animals	Per minutes
Young cattle, 1 year	27
Cattle, adult	12–16
Sheep, lamb	15–18
Sheep (adult)	12–15
Sheep (old)	9–12
Goat (kid)	12–20
Goat (adult)	12–15
Goat (old)	9–12
Pig	10–20
Dog, young	20–22
Mink	35–160
Silver fox	12–60
Rhesus monkey	15–30
Domestic fowl	15–30
Turkey	12–16
Pigeon	20–40
Duck	16–28
Goose	12–30
Camel	5–12
Whale	4–5

Symptoms of Heat in Cow

Symptoms	Intense heat	Intermediate	Weak heat
1. Excitement	Very much pronounced	Not pronounced	No excitement
2. Bellowing	Very often	Occasionally	Very seldom
3. Loss of appetite	Less appetite	Seldom less appetite	Normal
4. Peculiar movements of lumbosacral region	Generally appears	Sometimes appear	Rarely occur
5. Licking other animals	Always licks	Licks	Sometimes
6. *Mounting other animals	Always	Observed	Sometimes
7. Standing still when other cows or bulls try to mount	Always observed	Always	Common
8. Mucous from vulva	Common and generally copious in nature	Appears often	Very little appears and passes often unnoticed
9. Hypermia of vaginal mucous membranes	Pronounced	Not much	Difficult to detect
10. Swollen vulva	Very pronounced	Not much	Difficult to detect
11. Milk production	Less milk	Sometimes less	Normal

* Mounting word is used when an animal mounts (from behind) for sexual mating.

Reproductive Cycle of Domestic Animals

Species	Age of puberty	Nature of heat cycle recurrent	Duration of oestrous	Time of ovulation	Period of maximum fertility	Gestation period	Sperm survival in uterus
Cow	2–2.5 yrs	Polyestrous recurrence (21 days)	8–24 hrs average 19 hrs	14 hrs after the end of oestrus	Last 8 hrs of oestrous	282 days	20 hrs
Mare	2 yrs	Seasonally polyestrous (21 days)	3–40 days average 7 days	24 hrs before the end oestrous	Penultimate day of oestrous	336 days	2–3 days
Ewe	6–12 months	Seasonal	36 hrs	Later part of oestrous	2nd half of oestrous	150 days	22–42 hrs
Sow	5 months	Polyestrous	2–3 days	36 hrs after onset of oestrous and continues up to next 12 hrs	36 hrs after onset of oestrous	120 days	24 hrs
Bitch	9–12 months	Monoestrous	8 days (proper oestrous)	1–3 days after onset of oestrous proper	Next 3 days after the onset of oestrous	62 days	4 days
Buffalo	2.5 yrs bull 2yrs	Polyoestrous recurrence 21days	8 hrs – 3 days average 32 hrs	10–20 hrs up to the end of oestrous	Last 8 hrs of oestrous	307 days	Less than 24 hrs
Goat	4–8 months	Polyoestrous recurrence (18–27 days)	1–2 days	—	—	150 days	—
Camel	3–4 yrs	Polyoestrous recurrence (10–20 days)	1–7 days	—	—	406 days	—

Reproductive Cycle of Pet Animals

	Cats	Dogs	Guinea pigs	Hamsters	Mice	Rabbits
Age at puberty	6–15 months	6–12 months	55 to 70 days	5–8 weeks	35 days	5.5 to 8.5 months
Cycle type	Provoked ovulation seasonally polyoestrous spring and early fall 15–12 days	Monostrous all year, but mostly late winter and summer	Polyestrous	Polyestrous	Polyestrous	Polyestrous induced ovulation
Cycle length	15–21 days	6–7 month	16 days	4 days	4 days	1 month or more
Duration of heat	9–10 days in absence of male 4–6 days if mated	4–14 days standing heat	6–11 hrs	10–20 hrs	9–20 hrs	1 month or more
Best time for breeding	Daily from day 2 of heat	On alternate days from day 2 to end of heat	10 hrs after the start of heat	At the start of heat, 8–10 pm	At the start of heat	Anytime
First heat after birth	4–6 weeks	3–5 months	6–8 hrs	1–2 weeks after litter removed	2–4 days after litter removed	Immediate
Number of young	1–10	1–22	1–8	1–12	1–12	3–13

Chapter 27

Diamond News
for Veterinarians

▪ WHY SEMEN SORTING COULD REVOLUTIONISE DAIRY SECTOR

News by Akshay Varshney—November 22, 2016 (Dairy News of India)

Why semen sorting could revolutionise dairy sector

Cattle husbandry in the past was an activity aimed mainly to cater to the farming operations. But the utility of the cattle is *diminishing due to mechanisation*, and the objective of cattle keeping is progressively turning towards dairying.

As per the estimates, the contribution of the draft animals to India's total energy needs in the *farming sector has reduced from the levels of 71% in 1961 to 23.3% in 1991.* The declining trend continues and calls for production of more number of heifers. If, India has witnessed tremendous growth in dairy sector; it is mainly due to the growth in the crossbred population, which is growing at 7.6% annual rate.

Among the growing crossbred population, *males have almost no value or negative value* because of the declining need for draft animals coupled with the legal ban on cattle slaughter.

The crossbred male animals are eliminated either through early calf mortality due to neglect, or release into the village commons where they roam uncared for. The stray bulls become a nuisance due to the indiscriminate crossing and transmission of venereal diseases, and also cause damage and loss to farmers' crops and a significant loss of feed resources. The need of the hour is a technology that can boost production of crossbred heifers without generating unwanted males, is highly desired for building a profitable smallholder based dairy sector. The earliest research on semen sorting was done in the 1980s. This technology has been continually improving.

Sexed semen is assorted semen either containing X or Y chromosomes and the use of it *would produce the desired sex-male or female animal.* Semen sexing uses the principle of DNA concentration of X and Y chromosomes. X chromosomes contain 3.8% more DNA than Y chromosomes. The sorting of chromosomes (X or Y) is done using the flow–cytometer technology.

Semen sexing technology was introduced in the late 1990s in the domestic dairy industry. Under Rashtriya Krishi Vikas Yojana (RKVY), a pilot project has been taken up in Odisha for using 3, 138 doses of Jersey sexed semen procured from Viking Genetics, Denmark. Similarly, BAIF Development Research Foundation is also going to use sex-sorted semen in 25 high-performing Cattle Development Centres (CDCs) in five districts by March 2018. It is planned to use 5, 100 sex-sorted semen.

The sorted semen from HF pedigreed bull namely, Regancrest Tabber Benhart and Phil – RU Bogart Kronk ET and Tollenaars Mascoltea 718 ET with an average milk yield of more than 12, 500 kg per lactation will be used. Sorted semen from the Jersey pedigreed bulls, Wilsonview Jevon Magnum ET and GR Comsdale CC Celebrity Cindy ET with average milk yield of 10, 403 kg per lactation and 9, 566 kg per lactation respectively, will be used. These bulls have genetic merit to *produce cows to yield maximum 40 litres milk per day*. This intervention will help the state to benchmark the conception rate of sorted semen under different agroclimatic and socioeconomic conditions; and benchmark the conception rate of sorted semen in different categories of the cows like heifers and multiparous cows, of different localities; and to also benchmark the sexing ratio in the progeny produced from sorted semen usage. Use of sexed semen will result in the *birth of heifer calves 90% of the times* in contrast to non-sexed semen, which could result in the birth of female calves only in 50% of the times. Production of such genetically superior daughters will result in improving the desired traits in a shorter period, resulting in faster genetic progress. Use of sexed semen tends to produce more female calves, which biologically weigh less than the male calves and the percentages of difficult calving are reduced almost to half.

Cost Benefit

Reduced calving difficulties will help the cows to settle into milking quickly. The costs associated with handling difficult births and loss of calves could be reduced. The use of sexed semen will result in the elimination of the male calves right at the birth. This will result in the increased availability of feed and fodder resources. The overall reduction in the population will result in *less production of methane and other greenhouse gases* (GHGs) from livestock, which is a climate change mitigation measure.

The overall gain *from the use of sorted semen will be much higher compared to the use of frozen semen*. Our country needs to create own sex-sorted semen technology for the indigenous cow breeds like Gir, Rathi, Red Sindhi, Sahiwal, Binjharpuri and Haryana since the US companies have technology primarily for exotic cow breeds such as Holstein-Friesian and Jersey.

There are a large number of indigenous non-descript breedable cows; descript breedable cows and breedable she-buffaloes, and crossbreed breedable cows in the state. The crossbred produce nearly 41% of the milk and they are more productive than the indigenous cows.

There is scope for huge improvement in total yields of milk in the state from indigenous non-descript cows by using sorted semen of indigenous cow breeds Gir, Red Sindhi, Sahiwal, Binjharpuri and Haryana. Small to moderate use of female sexed semen will increase the supply of replacement heifers enough to satisfy the demand and in turn would have a significant impact. Using sexed semen will increase the supply of good dairy cows, leading to overall enhancement of milk production. All these efforts will make India's milk revolution sustainable in days to come.

ILLAWARRA BREED OF COWS (AUSTRALIA)

This is a wonderful news which can revolutionise Indian dairy industry and above all, can make crores of people living below poverty line win over poverty. It is deplorable that almost 99.9% of veterinarians and almost 100% of government high-ups have no knowledge of this cattle breed so suitable for India. We are still chasing Holsteins and Jersy cows of cold countries not suitable for India.

I am giving below the wonderful features of this Australian breed so that it may be brought to India for alleviation of poverty.
1. Illawarra produce milk in excess of 40 litres per day which has high protein and moderate fat and can support growing world demand for proteins.
2. Produce 40 litres in 300 days lactation.
3. It tolerates extremes of temperature from 0°C to over 40°C. Adapts well to varying climatic conditions.

4. Calving starts at 2 years age and regularly every 12 months.
5. Calving requires no help or attendance.
6. They can thrive on pasture based feeding system and are not housed any time of the year.
7. Lifetime total milk produced is more than 60,000 litres.
   One Illawarra cow can support one family (40 litres × ₹ 40 = ₹ 1600/day = ₹ 48,000 per month).

■ OSTRICH FARMING

Ostrich farming can be a very rich source of income in wastelands of India. One female ostrich produces about 110 eggs per year. Ostrich incubators are produced in India. One ostrich chick was sold (in Australia in 1995) at a cost of $5000. So, if 60 chicks are produced by one ostrich (wth 50% hatching), the income will be 300000 dollars per year. This comes to more than 1.5 crore per female ostrich. The cost of chicks may have come down but it is still a lucrative business. One ostrich produces about 3.5 meter of superior quality leather in the world. One pair of shoes of ostrich leather were sold in about the year 1995 for $900 (₹ 54000). Ostrich is also the best convertor of feed and can digest starch cellulose, hemicelluloses, etc. It hardly suffers from major infectious diseases. Hence, one ostrich can support about 100 Indian families with good income. India already has:
1. Good infrastructure for leather/shoe industry.
2. Wasteland to keep ostriches.
3. India produces incubators for ostrich eggs.
4. India has enough labour power for handling ostriches.

■ IMPROVED DESHI (VILLAGE FOWL) POULTRY

Indian villagers keep country poultry birds which do not require special housing and feeding but the villagers do not have knowledge of poultry vaccines which must be given for immunisation. Rural poultry farming has developed slowly but remarkably to produce 34,000 million eggs and 630 million broilers annually, contributing 11% of total poultry production. Galus, the red Indian jungle fowl and 'Aseel', the fighting type, are the baseline for more economical, disease resistant, stress-resistant egg and broiler breeds (Krishna B, Kayastha S, Dutta S and Roy PK 2010, Pashudhan, Sept issue). These evolved breeds give better results than traditional deshi birds and must be propagated by education and vaccination.

Indian Developed Rural Breeds

Vanjara, Giriraja, Gramapriya, and *Cari Golden* (developed by Central Avian Research Institute, Izzatnagar, UP).
   Vanjara produces 12–15 eggs per month.
   Cari Golden produces 15–20 eggs per month.
   Chicks are fed rice kani (broken rice) wheat kani, termites, etc. after 1 month age.

Advantages

1. These breeds are more colourful and attractive than village birds.
2. Can thrive in harsh weather, poor housing and management.
3. There is no broodiness.
4. Eggs and meat are more tasty, hence fetch better price.
5. There is less body fat.

6. Resistant to bacterial and viral diseases but vaccination ensures full safety. (Merek's Dis 0.2 ml SC at hatching La Sota 7th week (1 drop in eye) LaSota eyedrop 12th week, B2b 0.5 ml eyedrop, 16th week + deworming —monthly).

■ HYDROPONICS (LANDLESS CULTIVATION OF GREEN GRASS AND VEGETABLES WITH LEAST WATER REQUIREMENT AND WATER RECIRCULATION)

The population of India is exploding and the share of land for each person is getting less and less due to ever-expanding cities, villages, roads, factories and by saline water problem. Wasteland (unfit for agriculture) can also be used. About 2000 square feet of area can provide about 2 tonnes of lush green grass everyday. Total cost (on farm) comes to about ₹ 2.50 per kg. Grass can be grown in a rotation of 6–7 days providing daily greens. Cow urine in very small quantity acts as fertiliser. (Know how and equipment can be obtained from Chanakya Marg, Cozway Road, Tadwadi, Surat, Gujarat or from Vice-Chancellor, Jodhpur Agricultural University, Jodhpur). This method requires not much land, electricity, water or labour and only durable plastic trays, racks for trays and seeds are needed round the year. This method can provide green fodder for cows, calves, goats, sheep and even pigs.

Feeding these greens will also make animals safe from entry of diseases, poisoning from feed (nitrate, nitrite, HCN, etc.) parasites of animals and nutritional imbalance. All-round availability such as in rainy season, summer, long holidays like Deepawali, Holi, etc. is another big advantage.

Tellichery Goats

This breed of goats adapts itself to almost any climate, particularly dry, low rainfall due to climatic cnanges. It produces 1.5 to 2 litres of milk/day (with 150 to 200 days lactation period). Thus, 2–3 goats can provide best milk for a small family from a small housing space by feeding 300–400 g concentrate (costing about ₹ 10–12 per day). It produces 2–3 kids per kidding after about 5 months pregnancy.

This breed is reared in North Malabar, Tamil Nadu and Kerala. Weight of goats at 6 months is 20 to 24 kg and 40–50 kg in 12 months. Requirement for housing is simple, dry, comfortable (20 sq feet for buck, 15 sq feet for doe and 4 sq feet for kid) people in villages should give deworming injections PPR (vaccination is very cheap, once in a year) goat pox vaccine. Medicated water will prevent diarrhoea, the common cause of death of kids.

Goat Concentrate Mixture (kg of total)

Ingredient	For kid	Grower	adult
Maize	40	22	36
Gram chooni	10	20	5
Groundnut cake	22	35	16
Wheat bran	15	20	40
Mineral mixture	2.5	2.5	2.5
Salt	0.5	0.5	0.5
Vitamin mixture	25 g	25 g	10 g

Jhakrana Goats

This is one of the best goat breed for milk which produces 2–3 kg milk over a lactation period of 180–200 days, they are also prolific and produce twins in 40% deliveries and triplets are not uncommon. They are also good for meat. Average adult male is of 55 kg in weight and female is 45 kg in weight. Their skin is also superior and preferred for tanning. They are mainly found in Jhakrana and some adjoining villages of Behror of Alwar district of Rajasthan. They also withstand extremes of climate as in Rajasthan.

Boer Goats

This breed has been imported by some Indian dealers. It is a very big goat. The male attains about 90 kg and female 60 kg of weight. Most of the times twins or triplets are produced. It includes some genes of Indian breeds hence it is expected to survive well in India.

Jwongvi

This is a unique goat breed of China which survives on poor desert grasses and where rainfall is about 19 cm yearly. It produces world-class fur even at the age of 35 days.

For more details about goats contact Director Central Goat Research Institute, Maqudoom, District Mathura or Rural Agricultural Institute, Narayangaon, Maharashtra.

■ DISEASE PREVENTION PROGRAMME FOR GOATS

Goat farming is a profitable business and for providing good and easily digestible milk for children and old people but it has not become so popular due to less attention given to this 'poor man's cow'. I have experienced that goat rearing has failed as a goatery due to diseases and ignorance of the keepers about common disease preventive methods. In brief I suggest some vaccinations:

Months	Product	Adult goat	Kids	Source
January	CCPP	0.2–0.3 ml	0.2 ml	My own vaccine; not available commercially
April	HS (killed)	2–2.5 ml SC	0.2 ml SC	Any state government bio-products institute
Every 6 months	Enterotoxemia FMD + booster SC	See chapter on ET	See chapter on ET	Bovilis ET vaccine (MSD) or Cl perfringens vaccine inactivated (of MSD)
Goat pox		*See chapter on goat pox*		
Deworming	Ivermectin		1 ml per 50 kg BW SC	Endact LA of Vetoquinol and Endact Plus after 4–6 months
Medication (Preventive)				
Tiamutin	Oral medicine given soon on arrival of new goats for 3 days, 10–20 mg/kg BW, orally 5 days monthly (Galvoty of Intas)	Treatment 20–30 mg/kg BW for 3–5 days (CCPP)		5 kg plastic jar
Mineral mixture	Minshot (Intas) 1 ml/50 kg BW (up to 1 year); 1 ml/75 kg BW (1–2 years); 1 ml/100 kg BW (above 2 years) SC or deep IM	Once in 3–4 months		

Dosmin Forte (Merial —mix 1–2% in feed (regularly).
Bexoliv (syrup) of TTK 5–10 ml once daily every week.

INDEX/CONTACT DETAILS OF PHARMACEUTICAL COMPANIES
MENTIONED IN THIS MANUAL

Alembic Pharmaceuticals Limited
2nd Floor, Prime Corporate Park, Behind
ITC Grand Maratha Sheraton, Sahar Road,
Andheri East, Ashok Nagar, Andheri East,
Mumbai, Maharashtra 400099
Phone: 022-30611666/9829/9832
Email: alembic.foundation@alembic.co.in

Bovian Health Care Pvt. Ltd.
Vasavi Gold Stone, 2nd Floor, Survey No.
25, Near Military Football Ground,
Trimulgherry, Secunderabad-500 015,
Telangana.
Call Us +91-40-2799 0397/98
E-mail info@bovianhealthcare.com

Ayurvet Ltd.
6th floor Sagar Plaza,
District center, Laxmi Nagar, Vikas Marg
Delhi-110092
FAX: 011-22455991
e-mail: consumercare@ayurvet.com
Landline No: 011-22455993

G. Loucatos & Co.
Mercantile Chamber, 12, JN Heredia Rd,
Ballard Estate, Fort, Mumbai, Maharashtra
400001
Phone: 022 2261 8089
Fax : +91-22-2262 0786
E-mail : info@loucatos.com

Chembond Chemicals Limited
Chembond Centre
EL-71 Mahape MIDC,
Navi Mumbai 400 710, India.
Phone: +91 22 62643000; 022-39213001
Fax: +91 22 27681294
info@chembondindia.com

Kepler Vet Mission Pvt. Ltd.
"PARAS",7-Vidyanagar Society, Part-III,
Opp.Vidyanagar School,
Usmanpura, Ahmedabad – 380013,(Guj)
India.
Phone No. +91 79 30144400
Email ID: info@keplervet.com

Intervet India Pvt. Ltd.
(MSD Animal Health)
33, Pune-Nagar Road,
Viman Nagar,
Pune 411014
Phone no. +91 020 66294700/01
Fax no. +91 020 66050403

Pfizer Animal Health India Limited
Pfizer Centre, Patel Estate, Off S.V. Road,
Jogeshwari (W), Mumbai 400102
Tel: 022-66932000
Fax: 022-66797232; 09725352575
Email: girishkumar.rohit@pfizerindia.com

Vetoquinol India Animal Health Pvt. Ltd.
801, Sigma, 8th Floor,. Hiranandani
Business Park, Technology Street - Powai.
Mumbai, Maharashtra 400 076
Phone: 022-61322609
Email: consumerservicesindia@veto-
quinol.com

Zydus Animal Health
A division of Cadila Healthcare Ltd, is a
revered name in the ... Park, 5th Floor,
Satellite Cross Roads, Ahmedabad 380 015,
Gujarat
Tel: 91-79-26868681
Fax: 79-26868687
Email: enquiry@zydusahl.com

Pedigree
Mars International India Pvt. Ltd.
Survey No. 2099 - 2103,
Village Wargal, Siddipet Highway, Distt.
Medak 502279
Telangana, India
Email: pedigree.india@effem.com
Phone: Tel: 1800 407 11 21 21 (Toll free)
Mobile: +91 84523 06691/92

Van Vet Pvt. Ltd.
Shalin Complex, 1st Floor, Plot No 303, Rd
Number 5, Sector 22, Gandhinagar, Gujarat
382022
Phone: 079 2324 6501; 9375046501
Email: info@vanvet.co.in

Medisynth Naturals Pvt. Ltd.
1st Floor, Shivaji Mandir, N.C. Kelkar Road,
Dadar (W) , Mumbai,
Maharashtra,INDIA,400028
Tel: 022-32963295
Fax: 022-27686679
Email: sales@medisynth.com

TTK Healthcare Limited
Sreshtha Pinnacle # 39, Oliver Road
Mylapore, Chennai 600 004.
Email:hrd@ttkhealthcare.com
Phone: 846951511, 044-24980532,
42984444

Dosch Pharmaceuticals Pvt. Ltd.
Animal Health Division, BSEL Tech Park, B
Wing, 804, 8th Floor, Plot No 39/5 & 39/5
A, Vashi, Navi Mumbai 400703, Opposite
Vashi Railway Station
Phone : 02241149600, FAX: 022-41149616
Email: kaparmar@dosch.com,
info@dosch.com

Samarth Life Sciences Pvt. Ltd.
Samarth House, No. 168, Bangur Nagar
Goregaon West, Near Ayappa Temple,
Near Ayappa Temple, Goregaon West,
Mumbai 400090, Maharashtra
Phone: 08048026495, 022-28719501-09

Provimi Animal Nutrition Pvt Ltd
IS-40, KHB Industrial Area, Yelahanka
New Town, Bengaluru 560 064 Karnataka
Ph : +91 (0) 80-3368 0002 , 3368 0153
Fax : +91 (0) 80-2846 1520
Email : info@provimi.in,
customercare@cargill.com

Vetsfarma, Vets House
90-91, Urban Estate, Phase-1,
Jalandhar, Punjab, India
PIN – 144022
Phone: +91-181-435-3031-34
Email: vets@vetsfarma.com

HiMedia Bioscience
A-516, Swastik Disha Business Park, via
Vadhani Industrial Estate, L.B.S. Marg,
Mumbai, Maharashtra 400086
Phone: 022 6147 1919

Brihans Lab
Vaman Techno Centre, 7th Floor,
Makwana Road,
Off:Andheri-Kurla Road,
Marol Naka, Andheri (East)
Mumbai 400059.
Phone No: 022- 42300800
Email: info@brihans.in

Hester Biosciences Ltd
Pushpak 1st floor
Motilal Hirabhai Road
Panchvati Circle, Ahmedabad
Gujarat 380006, India
Phone: +91 79 2644 5106, +91 79 2644 5107
Fax: +91 79 2644 5105
Email: mail@hester.in

Intas Animal Health
4th Floor, Premier House, Opp.
Gurudwara
Sarkhej-Gandhinagar Highway
Ahmedabad 380054. Gujarat. India
Email: iah@intaspharma.com
Fax: +91 (22) 6646 6196
Tel: +91 (79) 6652 366

Indian Immunologicals Ltd.
Road No. 44, Jubilee Hills,
Hyderabad 500033 Telangana, India.
Tel: +91 8466924444, Tel: +91 7997915555,
Tel: 040-67682200
Email: info@indimmune.com

Tineta Pharma Pvt. Ltd.
G-15/16, Solaris II, Saki Vihar Road,
Manohar Nagar, Marol, Powai,
Mumbai, MH 400072
Call Us:– 022 2847 1611
Email: tineta@tineta.com

Merial Animal Health
Sanofi House, CTS No.117-B, L&T Business
Park, Saki Vihar Road, Powai, Mumbai,
Maharashtra 400072
Phone: 022 3070 7800

Neospark
Drugs and Chemicals Private Limited
Corporate Center,
241, B.L. Bagh, Panjagutta,

Hyderabad 500 082, Telangana, India.
Phone: 91-40-49012345 (30 lines)
E-mail: mail@neospark.co.in
URL: http://www.neospark.com

Natural Remedies
Plot No. 5B
Veerasandra Industrial Area, 19th K.M. Stone
Hosur Road, Electronic City
Bangalore, Karnataka
India 560 100
Email: sales@naturalremedy.com

Virbac Animal Health India Pvt. Ltd.
604, 6th floor, Western Edge – I
Magathane - Western Express Highway
Borivali (East) - Mumbai 400 066
Telephone –022–4008 1333
Fax - 022-40081300

Vetina Distributors LLP
401-B, Town Square
Viman Nagar
Pune, India 411014
Email ID : customerservice@vetina.com
Phone No. : (020) 2663 3615

Vet Mankind Pharma Ltd.
208, Okhla Industrial Estate,
Phase III, New Delhi 110020
Ph.: (+91)-11-46541111 (30 Lines),
Fax: (+91)-11-46541382
Website: www.mankindpharma.com
Email: contact@mankindpharma.com
businessdevelopment@mankindpharma.com
Ph: (+91)-11-46541111, 46541400
Fax: 011-46541382

Carus Laboratories Pvt. Ltd.
Menu; Plot No 75, Sector-3, HSIIDC, Karnal
132001, Haryana, India. Phone :91-184-
2220565
Email: caruslabs@gmail.com

The Himalaya Drug Company
Makali, Bengaluru, KA, 562 162, India
Phone: 1(800) 208-1930/1(800) 425-1930
080-67549999 (Toll-free in India)
Email: ustomer.service@himalayawellness
.com

Eldin Pharma (Vet)
B-G/80, Sardar Patel Complex, Sidhpur
Char Rasta, Patan, Gujarat 384265, India
Phone: 917874165503, 9723912134

Lyka Animal Healthcare Division
101, Shiv Shakti Industrial Estate, Opposite
to Mittal Estate, Andheri Kurla Road
Andheri (East)
Mumbai 400059
Email: info@lykaahd.com
Phone: 022-66112200
Fax: 91 22 6611 2225

Polchem Hygiene Laboratories Pvt. Ltd.
6 Sr No 28 Gandharva Apts, Off Karve Rd
Erandwane, Pune - 411004, Nr Mehendale
Garage Opp Hotel Abhishek
Phone: 020-25439858/74
Fax: 020-25439789
Email: polchem@vsnl.com

Venky's
3/303, 3rd Floor, Sharda Centre, 11/1
Erandwane, Pune 411004
Phone: +91-20-24251530 to 41
Fax: +91-20-24251077
Email: response@venkys.com

Medisynth
D-282, M.I.D.C, Turbhe, Navi Mumbai
Maharashtra 400705
Phone: 022 2768 1116
Email: info@medisynth.com
Royal Canin (Veterinary diet),
Email: feedback.india@royalcanin.com

CLASSIFIED INDEX OF MEDICINES

Antibiotics

Lyka Exports Ltd			
Ampillin injection (IM, IV)	Ampicillin	2.5 g	All systemic bacteria infections; dose 5/10 mg/kg BW
Baxivet D injection (IM, IV)	Ampicillin + dicloxacillin	2.5 & 4 g	10 mg/kg BW twice in a day
Seft plus injection (IM, IV)	Seftriaxone sod. Salbactum	3–5 g	5–10 mg kg BW twice a day
Lyfovet injection (IM, IV)	Sephotoxim sod.	4 g	10 mg/kg (IM, IV)
Lykaseft vet (IM, IV) Small: 10–15 mg/kg BW	Seftrioxone	3 g	Large Animal 5–10 mg/kg BW
Lykacetin (IM, IV)	Chloramphenicol	1, 2, 3 g vial	Large 2–4 mg/kg IV 20–30 mg/kg BW IM Small: 30–40 mg/kg /IM 10 mg kg BW IV
Lykadin oral	Sulfadimidine	4 bolus × 10	Large: 1–2 bolus/50 kg BW; half bolus after 1 day
Lyramycin	Gentamicin, wounds, surgery, prolapse	50 & 100 g paste	External application

Antimicrobial

Zydus Animal Health		
Dicrysticine injections Dicrysticine DS (double contents)	Streptomycin procain penicillin diluents 7.5 ml	2 ml/50 kg BW 1 ml/5 kg BW (small animal)
FPP injection (FPP 20 and FPP 40)	Fortified procain penicillin + penicillin G. Sod 5 ml dist. water	400 units/kg BW/ 24 hrs small animals 200000–400000 24 hrs/IM
Penicillin G procaine in oil—use 14 gauze needle	Procain pen G	Large: 8000 IU/kg BW Dogs, cats, 2 lakh 4 lakh/3 days
Vet Clox Forte injection	Ampicillin sod., Cloxacillin sod. 10 ml dist. water	5–10 /kg BW 24 hours 3–5 days 1–2 m/25 kg BW (large)
Steclin inj	Oxytetracyclin	1–2 ml/10 kg BW. IM, IV, SC
Oxytetracyclin (long-acting) Not for horses, dogs, and cats	200 mg/ml	20 mg/kg BW (1 ml/10 kg) Single shot IM/72 hours
Enrodac 10 inj	100 mg/ml Enrofloxacin	1 ml/20 kg BW IM, IV 3–5 days. Salmonella— 7–10 days
Vetazo inj	Caffrioxone sod	

· Cadila Pharmaceuticals		
Enrotreat inj	Enrofloxacin 10%	2.5 mg/kg BW
Trepin inj	Centrimoxazole inj	Large animal — 15–30 ml daily; small animal 2–5 ml daily Dose: 2–5 mg/kg BW IM, IV, or SC inj

Note: In this drug index it is not possible to include all drugs for all conditions hence important and tried drugs are included so that a doctor may select *vis-à-vis* availability in market. Other medicines are already mentioned in the text.

Antibiotics Vetoquinol Co

Name	Contents	Packing	Dose
Mastiwok	Cefoperazone sodium	10 ml	Single dose, intramammary
Tilox	Ampicillin sod; cloxacillin sod	5	One time
Wocef	Ceftriaxone	3 g, 4 g	5–10 mg/kg BW; IM, IV
Wocef-XP	Ceftriaxone Tazobactam Ceftiofur Sodium	3.375 g 4.5 g 1 g	5–10 mg/kg BW IM, IV route
Wofor	Ceftiofur sodium	1 g	1.1–2.2 mg/kg , IM route
Vetocyclin-DS	Oxytetracycline Dinydrate Oxytcracycline	30 ml and 100 ml	5–10 mg/kg IM, IV, route
Meriquin injection	Enrofloxacin 100 mg benzyl alcohol	100 ml	2.5 mg/kg BW; 1 ml/40 kg BW IM, EV, SC, route
Meriflox injection	Levofloxacin	15 ml and 50 ml	5 ml/100 kg IM, IV route

Other Antibiotics

Name of drug	Dose	Trade name with presentation
Gentamicin (40 mg/ml) (aminoclycoside)	All animals: 4–5 mg/ kg BW BID IM, IV	Inj. Gentamicin 30 and 100 ml (KAPL, TTK) Inj. Ranbamycin 100 ml Inj. Microgenta (80 mg/ml) 100 ml
Amikacin (250 mg/ml) (aminoglycoside)	D/cat: 10 mg/kg BW TID IM, IV, SC	Inj. Tamik…50 ml, 100 ml (TTK) Inj. Amikin 30 ml, 100 ml (Vetsfarma) Inj. Amidac…10 ml, 50 ml, 100 ml (Zydus)
Kenamicin (aminoglycoside)	C/B: 5–10 mg/kg BW D/cat: 5 mg/kg BW IM, IV	Inj. Kancin (250 mg/ml)… 50 ml (Morvel) Inj. Kancin 0.5 g, 1 g (Alembic)

Product	Composition	Indications	Dosage
Mofoi	Each ml contains: Moxifloxacin— 100 mg	*Respiratory infection:* Pneumonia Bronchopneumonia Contagious Bovine Pleuro Pneumonia (CBPP) *Mammary Infection:* Mastitis *Uterine infection:* Metritis, Endometritis, Pyometra, Retained Placenta	5 mg/kg BW by IM/IV route
Sulbian	Each vial contains: Ceftriaxone 3 g Sulbactam 1.5 g	*Mammary infection:* Mastitis *Uterine infection:* Metritis, Pyometra Retained Placenta Uterine Prolapse	10 mg/kg BW by IM/IV route
Bactogon	Each vial contains: Ceftriaxone 3 g	Pneumonia Bronchopneumonia Haemorrhagic Septicemia Metritis, Endometritis Pyometra and Mastitis	5–10 mg/kg BW by IM/IV route
Bovixin LA*	Each ml contains: Oxytetracycline Dihydrate I.P. Equivalent to anhydrous Oxytetracyclime 200 mg 2-pyrrolidone-vehicle system QS	*Bacterial infection:* Metritis Endometritis, Pyometra, HS BQ, Mastitis, Pneumonia Calf scour, Enteritis, Joint ill, Navel ill, CCPP Leptospirosis, Wooden Tongue, Foot rot, Wounds and Surgical conditions Secondary bacterial infections *Protozoal infection:* Amoebiasis, Anaplasmosis and Coccidiosis *Rickettsial infection* *Chlamydial infection*	20 mg/kg BW by deep IM injection
Durocin DS	Each ml contains: Enrofloxacin 200 mg Bromhexine HCl 15 mg	Respiratory Tract infection GI tract infection, urinary tract infection, skin and soft tissue infection, mixed bacterial and Mycoplasma infections	1 ml per 20 kg BW

*LA = Long-acting for 72 hours.

Antibiotics (Virbac)

Name	Contents	Pack	Dose
Amoxyrum (tabs)	Amoxicillin	2 tab	1 tablet/200 kg BW Fever, pneumonia
Amoxyrum Forte injection	Amoxicillin + Sulbactam	300 mg vial 3000 mg 4500 m	7–10 mg/kg BW IM, IV or intramammary for Mastitis, etc.

Fortivir injection LA	Enrofloxacin	30 ml vial	3 ml/40 kg BW repeat at 72 hrs IM, IV, SC; 2–3 sites
Lixen (oral)	Cephalexin	1.5 g tab	1 tab/150 kg BW
Lixen IU intrauterine suspension	Cephalexin	1.5 g/60 ml (4 g bottle)	4 g in 60 ml intrauterine infections
Trox powder	Tylosin tart 50 %	120 g bottle	1 g per litre drinking water (Mycoplasma inf.)

Antibiotics (Hester Biosciences)

CuR injection (IM only) 30 ml and 100 ml	As for Fortivir above	Injection 30 ml/400 kg BW
Chek B injection (IM/IV/SC) 4 g + 20 ml water	All routine infections	Cow etc : 5–10 mg/kg BW
ICEFT 1000 injection (IM) 1000 mg	Respiratyory +reproductive+ hoof	1.1 to 2.2 mg/kg BW, IM

Antibiotics of Mankind Vet

Moxikind-Clav 3.6	Amoxicillin + Clavulinic acid, mastitis	3.6 g vial dose 10 mg/kg BW IM/IV
Enrostrong PZ injection	Enrotloxacin + Pefloxacin + Zinc (mainly, *E. coli*, mastitis, pneumonia, diarrhoea, etc.)	Dose 1 vial injection/day/ 3–5 days

Antibiotics of MSD

1. *Floxidin LA (single dose):* 50 ml injection for IM/SC use; dose 7.5 to 12.5 mg/kg BW; works for 48 to 72 hours.
2. *Cobactan:* Cefoquinome injection. Very good for Pasteurella of all types and *E. coli*, mastitis.
3. *Floxidin vet:* Injection, once daily for 3–5 days; 15 ml and 50 ml vials.

Antibiotics of Merial

1. *Seftifur sod.:* 1 g injection; dose 1.1 –2.2 mg/kg, IM or SC ; 3–5 days.
2. *Safevet Forte:* Ceftriaxone and salbactam, 3, 4.5, and 7.5 g IM, IV, or SC; 5–10 mg/kg (mastitis).
3. Safevet injection—3 g vial.
4. *Clampivet-S:* Ampicillin and salbactam injection; 100 ml vial, IM/SC 7.5–12.5 mg/kg; repeat at 48–72 hours.

Intas (Nuvo) division of Animal Health—Antimicrobials

Name	Contents	Dosage	Packing
Intacef Tazo IM/IV injection	Ceftriaxone 500 mg, Tazobactam 62.5 mg	Dog, cat: 15–25 mg/kg BW daily for 3–5 days; also H.S, pneumonia, mastitis metritis, etc.	562.5 mg vial
Intacef Pet IM/IV injection	Ceftriazone 500 mg	Bronchopneumonia, cystitis, UTI, metritis, etc; dose as above	500 mg vial

Contd...

Name	Contents	Dosage	Packing
CEF-PET tab	Cefpodoxime	UTI, skin, GI infections, wounds, abscess, etc. 5–10 mg/kg BW orally once/day	100 mg tab × 10
Flobac SA, injection, IM/SC/IV slow	Enrofloxacin 100 mg/ml	As above + CCPP, etc.	30 ml, 50 ml, and 100 ml vials
Intamox injection IM/IV	Amoxicillin Cloxacillin	As above + leptospirosis; Bovines: 6–10 mg/kg BW	2.5, 3.5, and 4.5 g vials
Intamox-O bolus 1.5 g	Amoxicillin	As for Intamox Dose-1 bolus/200 kg BW for 3–5 days	Strips of 2 boli
Intacef injection, IM/IV	Ceftriaxone	As Intaceph above Dose: bovine: 5–10 mg/kg BW; calf, sheep, goat: 10–15 mg/kg; dog, cat: 15–25 mg/kg BW for 3–5 days	250, 500, 1000 mg vials 2, 3, 4 g vials
Intacef Tazo IM, IV injection	Ceftriaxone and Tazobactam	Dose as for Intacef injection	562.5, 2250 mg, 3375, 4500 mg
Xyrofur injection, SC	Respiratory, reproductive, skin, foot rot infections, UTI	Dose: cattle, sheep, etc. 1.1 to 2.2 mg/kg BW; buffalo: 2.2–4.4 mg/kg BW	1 g vial
Zoctim injection, IM, IV; Ceftizoxime LA	Mastitis Ceftizoxime	Dose: bovine 5–10 mg/kg BW; repeat before 96 hours	1.5 and 2.5 g vial
AC-Vet Forte injection, IV, IM	Ampicillin Cloxacillin	Livestock dose: 6–10 mg/kg BW for 3–5 days	3g
AC-Vet Macx	As above	As above	4.5 g
Alembic Antibiotics			
Aldin-L (oral)	Neomycin + Bismuch subsalicylate	GI tract infections Dose: 1 bolus/100 kg BW, twice daily for 2–3 days	4 boli
Bacipen injection IM, IV	Ampicillin sod.	GI tract infections 5–10 mg/kg BW	2–2.5 g
Enrox injection IM, IV	Enrofloxacin 100 mg/ml	GI, respiratory infections Mycoplasma, UTI Dose: 2.5–5 mg/kg BW	15 and 100 ml
MCEFT injection IV only	Ceftizoxime	Clinical/subclinical mastitis Dose: 5 mg/kg BW	1.5, 2.5, 3 g vials
MAMA L-AZ infusion of udder	Azithromycin and Neomycin	Mastitis and Dry Cow therapy	5 g disposable syringe
Moxel , IM, IV injection	Amoxicillin + Cloxacillin	Respiratory and GI infections Dose: 10 mg/kg/BW 3–5 days	
Xceft injection, IM	Ceftiofur sod	Indications: as for Xyrofur	

■ ANTI-INFLAMMATORY/PAINKILLERS/ ANTIPYRETICS

Alembic

Aletol, injection—Tolfenansic acid, IM.

Ketop: Ketoprofen 100 mg/1 ml, IM/IV, 3–5 days.

Melambic: Meloxicam 5 mg/1 ml, IM/IV (cattle, sheep, goat, dogs, pig).

Melambic P: Meloxicam + paracetamol + Lignocaine—30 and 100 ml vials (all species) Inj.
Melambic P bolus (oral).

Cargil Incorporated

Polygesic	Nimesulide + Pitofenon: injection	dose: 2–4 mg/kg BW, IM, 30 and 100 ml
Pyridase	Nimesulide + Paracetamol bolus	dose: large animal: 2 boli, 2 times a day; small animal, 1 bolus 2 times a day

Vets Pharma

Meloxi plus injection	Meloxicam + Paracetamol	dose: 1 ml/10 kg BW, 30 and 100 ml
Meloxi injection	Meloxicam	30 and 100

Intas (Neovet)

Maxxtol injection: Tolfenamic acid/40 mg/ml; dose: cattle, etc: 4 mg/kg BW, IM or IV.

Melonex Z Plus: Meloxicam, Paracetamol and Serratiopeptidase (reduces swelling), dose: 1 bolus per 250 kg BW, daily.

Melonex Power injeciton: Meloxicam and Lignocaine, dose: 2.5 ml /100 kg BW, prolapse, mastitis, etc.

Melonex Plus bolus: Meloxicam and Paracetamol; dose: large: 1 bolus /200 kg BW, daily.

MSD

Vetalgin injection (33 ml): Analgin+ Chlorbutol (bacteriostat); dose: horse: 20–60 ml; cattle: 20–40 ml; sheep, goat: 2–8 ml, IV or IM injection.

Unixin (Hester): For pain, fever, colic (Meglumine), IV/IM injection; .2 mg/kg BW.

Merial

Vet Profen 100 ml injection: Ketoprofen pyrexia, pain, fever; dose: 2–4 mg/kg/BW.

Vetoquinol

Tolfine injection: Tolfenamic acid (NSAID); dose: cattle: 1 ml/kg BW; dog, cat: 4 mg/kg BW, SC or IM injection.

Proxyvet-MP: Meloxycam + Paracetamol; dose: 30 ml/300 kg BW, IM injection.

Virbac

Inflavet Plus tab: Like Melonex powder, see catalogue of Virbac for dose.

Inflavet injection

Megludyne 20 ml injection: Flunixin Meglamine; dose: 2 ml/45 kg BW; dogs: 1 ml/kg BW, IM or slow IV injection.

Karpofen (Zydus): 10 and 30 ml single dose (IM, IV, SC injection); dose: cattle: 1.4 mg/kg; horse:0.7 mg/kg; 65 hours half-life.

NASAIDs

Zydus

Flunimeg injection—Flunixin meglumine (as Megludyn above).

Oxalgin-NP bolus—Nimesulide + Paracetamol.

Oxalgin injection—Nimesulide 100 mg/ml.

Zobid-M injection —Meloxicam.

Zobid-M—Meloxicam bolus.

Esgipyrin N injection—Phenylbutazone, analgin + lignocain—deep IM injection; large animal: 5–15 ml; small animal: 1–5 ml.

▓ CORTICOSTEROIDS

Isoflud injection—Isoflupredone			5 –10 ml injection.
Dexona injection—Dexamethasone	5 ml	0.5–1 ml/10 kg BW.
Vetalog injection—Triamcinolone	5 ml	0.1–0.2 mg/kg BW.

▓ INTRAMAMMARY INFUSIONS

Zydus

Uddercef 3.5 g Cefuroxime sod. 250 mg	1 syringe infused perquarter for 3 milkings
pendistrin penicillin, streptomycin sulfamerazine, cortisone	1 tube per quarter, 12 hourly, 1–6 times
Vetclox Plus 10 ml tube—Cloxacillin, ampicillin	3 tubes per quarter, then 1 tube per quarter, 24 hourly

Neovet/Intas

Mammicef	Cephoparazone 250 mg = 10 ml syringe	Infuse 1 syringe per quarter
Mammitel	Colistin sulphate + Cloxacillin	Infuse 1 syringe per quarter 12 hourly
MSD		
Cobactan LC	75 mg Cetquinome per syringe (box of 3)	Infuse 12 hourly
Vetoquinol		
Mastiwok	Cefoperazone 250 mg in 10 ml syringe	Infuse 12 hourly
Alembic		
Mamal-AZ	Azithromycin and neomycin—5 g syringe	Infuse 1 syringe per quarter

▓ MAGGOTED WOUNDS SPRAY

1. D Mag spray (Neovet/Intas).
2. Dos spray (Merial): 100 ml herbal spray.

3. Bovispray (Bovian Health Care).
4. *Skin care (Globion India Pvt Ltd):* 100 ml spray for maggots, mange, fungus, and surgical cases.
5. Zymagout (Zydus): herbal, 40 and 100 ml.
6. Topicure spray (Natural Remedies).

ANTIALLERGIC DRUGS

1. *Avilin injection (MSD):* IM, IV, injection (Chlorpheniramine); dose as Anistamin.
2. *Cadistin injection (Zydus):* Chlorpheniramine): Large animal: 3–5 ml, IM, small animal: 0.5–1 ml.
3. *Anistamin injection (Neovet/Intas):* Chlorpheniramine, 100 ml vial; dose: large animal 5–10 ml/IM; small animal 1–2 ml.
4. *Bovistamine IM injection (Bovian healthcare):* Chlorpheniramine): 30 and 100 ml; dose 1 ml/20 kg BW.
5. Lorfen injection IM (Vets Pharma); Chlorpheniramin; 100 ml vial, dose as for Anistamin.
6. Avil vet (Merial) injection, 10 ml and 100 ml: Dose: large animals 5–10 ml IM; small animal 1–3 ml IM.

SEDATIVES (LOCAL/GENERAL ANAESTHESIA)

1. *Siquil injection (Zydus):* Triflupromazine hydrochloride 5 ml vial; dose: 1–2 mg/kg BW. It also helps milk let down.
2. *Flumimeg (Zydus) 10 ml injection IM/IV:* Analgesic, anticolic; dose: 1–2 ml/45 kg BW; horse: 1 ml/45 kg BW; dog 0.5–1 ml.
3. *Spasmovet injection IM (Vetoquinol):* Diclomine hydrochloride, 30 ml vial; relief of spasm, pain, colic, biliary colic; 1 ml/20 kg BW.
4. *Unixin IV, IM injection (Hester):* Flunixin meglumine; dose: 1.1–2.2 mg/kg BW; analgesic, anticolic; 20 ml vial.
5. Spasmovet (Vetoquinol) injection 30 ml; contains diclomine hydrochloride 10 mg per ml; for renal, biliary, intestinal colic, spasms of uterus, sedative after removal of placenta; Dose: 1 ml/20 kg BW or 10–20 ml in large animals; 0.5 to 2 ml in dogs.
6. *SPAS (G. Loucatos Co):* IM injection of diclomine hydrochloride, 30 ml vial relieves GI spasms, pain colic, urinary colic, rectal prolapsed, antiemetic in simple stomach anaimals; dose: cattle and horses 10–15 ml; sheep an goats 1–2 ml; dogs 0.5–1 ml.

RUMENOTORICS

1. *Bovirum bolus (Zydus):* Blisters of 4 boli.
   Dose: cattle 3–4 boli daily.
2. *Rumobuff (Merial product):* Buffer fortified with live yeast; prevents rumen acidosis, fibre digestion, prevents laminitis.
3. *Kepatite bolus (Kepler):* Blister of 4 boli; contains live yeast on herbal rumen stimulants.
4. *Rumeric injection (Virbac);* For rumen and liver dysfunction; has major amino acids; dose: 1 ml/kg BW for 3–5 days.
5. *Rumen FS (Alembic):* Mineral, yeast, enzymes for rumen indigestion; strips of 4 boli, 2 boli twice a day for 5 days.

6. *Rumicell (Bovian Health):* Dose: 2 boli BD for 3–4 days.
7. *Rumentas (Bovicura/Intas):* Ant. Pot. Tartrate, iron, copper and cobalt; strips of 4 boli.
8. *Floratone bolus and Floratone Forte bolus (Concept product):* 3 × 1 and 4 × 1 strips of bolus.
9. *Biobloom powder (Zydus):* Saccharomyces lactobacillus and 4 enzymes; 250 g and 1 kg packets.
10. *Bovilax:* Rumenotoric powder, 250 g and 500 g.
11. *Ecotas bolus (Bovicura):* Strips of 8 boli.

▇ RUMEN BYPASS (PROTEINS, FATS AND MINERALS)

1. *Zydus:* Fat Milk Dhara powder: Bypass protein and fat; 1 kg and 2 kg packs.
2. *Fat Plus powder (Virbac product):* Optimises milk fat and rumen pH.
3. *Khurak (Alembic):* Bypass proteins, minerals and probiotics, 300 g, 1.5 kg and 15 kg.
4. *Kalori powder (Merial):* High digestibility 95% fat, fat 80–84%, calcium 8–12% package, 1, 5, and 25 kg.
5. *Lacto-four (Chembond Chemicals):* Bypass protein, fat, vitamins, probiotics; cow 50 g/day, sheep/goat: 5–7 g/day; 1 and 5 kg pack.
6. *Cafplan (Bovicura/Intas):* Bypass protein, fat, yeast, and minerals; 3 kg jar.
7. *HFM:* Chelated bypass protein, carbohydrates and fat with chromium 1 kg and 20 kg.
8. *Milk Dhara (Zydus):* Bypass fat, protein, carbohydrates, chelated chromium and probiotics. Dose: Cows, etc. 100 g daily or 1 to 1.5% of feed.
9. *Galacshot (Cargil):* Bypass fat, glycogenic and lipogenic substances and probiotics; dose 100 g/day/animal.

▇ VITAMINS

Zydus

Belamyl injection (also contains liver extract).

Neuroxin M: Methylcobalamin and nicotinamide injection.

Vitakey injection (multivitamin injection, 11 ingredients).

Vetade injection (Vitamin A, D_3, and E).

Merial

Gold Boost injection: All B vitamins + liver extract.

Health Up: 200 ml vitamins, zinc, iron containing oral tonic.

Virbac

Brotone (oral): 120, 200, 500 ml; 2 and 5 litre jars yeast extract, liver extract, nicotinic acid.

Kepler

Petmina tablets: Vitamins and minerals.

Cargil

Nutria-sacc; Vitamin A, D_3, E, B_3, and all minerals; 1, 5, and 25 kg.

KEMFED WP (Chembond): All vitamins, minerals, by pass, probiotics (28 items).

Vets Pharma

B Jet injection: Multi B vitamin injection, 100 ml.

Brihans

1. *B-Liv 100:* Oral, liver extract, B_{12}, methionine, choline, etc; 200 ml, 500 ml, 1 litre, and 5 litre.
2. *Brimix:* Powder premis; Vitamin, A, D_3, E, K, all B vitamins, calcium, folic acid, yeast and choline; 5 kg and 25 kg bags; mix 250 g/tonne feed.

▇ DRUGS FOR ANAEMIA

1. Ferrites injection (Intas)—10 ml injection.
2. Ferrimin syrup (Ektek Pharma) 200 ml.
3. Ferritas bolus (Intas) 5 × 1 pkt.
4. *Livoferol:* for Ruminants—liver, iron, thiamin, riboflavin, nicotinamide; 500 ml, 1 and 5 litre.
5. RBC liquid (Vetoquinol) 200, 500 ml.
6. Liverton liquid (Neospark): Iron, copper, cobalt, B_{12}, selenium, tricholine and herbs; 500 ml, 1 and 5 litre.
7. Tribivet injection (Intas).
8. Tribivet M injection.
9. *Healthup PRO:* Oral for pets, 200 ml bottle.
10. *Rumentas:* Iron, copper, cobalt, strips fo 4 boli for cattle.
11. *KNZ tricks:* Iron, zinc, iodine, magnesium, lick for ruminants.
12. *Sharkoferrol (Alembic):* Malted, tasty, oral liquid, 300 mg iron, 100 mg copper, 1.5 mg cobalt, 15 mcg cyanocobalamine; dose: cow, etc. 30–50 g/animal/day; small animals 10–15 g/day; packing: 450 g and 2.25 kg.
13. *Rumen F.S. (Alembic):* Dose: 2 boli per day/5 days (Box 15 strips × 4 boli).

▇ ANTI-BLOOD PROTOZOAL DRUGS

1. *Surral (Alembic):* Contains isometamidium chloride HCl: 250 mg/vial.
2. *Nilbery (Neovet/Intas):* For Trypanosoma, Babesia, and mixed infection and Pyrexia of unknown origin. Contains Diminazine Diaceturate; 30 ml bottle; dose: 3.5–7 mg/kg BW.
3. *Berenil 7% RTU (MSD):* Treats babesiosis, trypanosomiasis, theileriasis, mixed infections and PUO. Contains Diminazine aceturate; dose: 5–10 ml/100 kg BW, resistant trypanosomes 10 ml/100 kg BW; also give 3–4 antibiotic injections on alternate days. Packing: 20, 30, and 90 ml.
4. *Batrynil (Zydus):* Diminazine aceturate injection; indications and dose as for Berenil.
5. *Prozomin injection (Virbac):* Contains Diminazine. Indications, dose, etc. as for Berenil. Presentation 30 ml RTU.

6. *Antrycid (Virbac) injection:* For prevention and treatment of trypanosomiasis. Contains Quinapyramine Sulphate, dissolve in 15 ml distilled water. SC injection at the rate of 2 ml per 45 kg BW.

7. *Triquin and Triquin 5 (Vetoquinol):* For treatment of trypanosomiasis (Surra); 2.5 g with sterile water to dissolve quinapyramine sulphate in 15 ml distilled water. Inject 3 ml per 100 kg BW, SC.

8. *Zokil (RTU, Mankind product) injection:* Diminazine 30 ml and 90 ml dose as for Berenil.

9. *Nyzom injection:* 250 mg Isometamidium HCl with sterile water for injection. For treatment of trypanosomiasis. Inject 0.25–0.5 mg/kg BW. Double dose for prevention. Dog 1 mg/kg BW by deep IM injection.

10. *Zubion (Intas):* Contains Buparvaquone for treatment of theileriosis. Inject 1 ml/ 20 kg BW by IM route. Repeat within 48–72 hours, if necessary.

11. *Bupaven injection (Venky) 20 ml:* Dose as for Zubion.

12. *Trityl (RTU injection):* Contains Diminazone aceturate 70 mg and phenazone 375 mg. Treats babesiosis, trypanosomiasis, theileriosis and PUO. Dose 1 ml/ 10–20 kg BW, IM.

13. IMIZET injection treats Babesia, Ehrlichia and Anaplasma by two injections 2 weeks apart (Intas product).

◼ IMPORTANT PERFORMANCE ENHANCERS (FOR MILK)

1. *Goldboost injection (Merial):* Anorexia, improving appetite; Sheep, goats: 0.5 to 1.0 ml dose; cattle: 3–5 ml IM/ 2–3 days.

2. *Doscal M injection:* Preventing Ca and magnesium deficiency in high yielding cows, grass tetany; 1 ml/kg BW, slow IV, SC.

3. *Govidha granules (Kepler):* For fat, SNF, and milk quantity; oral dose: Cows: 30 g daily; goats 15 g daily + more greens + 250 g concentrate.

4. *Lactoboon tablets (Lyka):* Orally 5–10 tablets daily.

5. *Casphodil Gold suspension (Lyka):* Cows, etc. 100 ml daily.

6. *Vetomin S (Vetoquinol):* Chelated minerals; cows, etc. 30–40 g daily.

7. *Biovet-YC (Vetoquinol):* Cows, etc. 15–20 g/day; goat, etc. 5–10 g/orally/day.

8. *Overmet (Vetoquionol):* 10 g/day orally or 1 kg/tonne feed in cows, etc.

9. *Wokagest (Vetoquinol):* Digestibooster; cows, etc. 2 boli daily, goat, etc. bolus.

10. *MP Power (Bovian Health):* 50–100 g/day; cow, etc. orally.

11. *Boostmin (Bovian Health):* 30–50 g/cow/day, orally.

12. *Nubo (Bovian):* 30–60 g/cow/day, orally.

13. *Nubo High (Bovian):* 50–100 g/buffalo/day up to 8 litre milk and 6 g/litre/day for more milk.

14. *Otiblend (Bovian):* Liquid tonic; 10 ml per 100 kg BW for 5–7 days.

15. *Amunity (Virbac):* Immunity booster; buffaloes/cows: 25 g daily.

16. *Agrimin Forte (Virbac) powder:* Cows, etc. 50 g/daily; goats, etc. 5–10 g/day.

17. *Chelated Agrimin Forte (Virbac):* Same dose, etc. as for Agrimin Forte. Loss of minerals very low due to chelation.

18. *Equimin (Virbac) powder for horses:* Dose 100 g daily, foals: 150 g/day.

19. *Fat Plus (Virbac):* Powder for high fat and SNF; good for rumen and digestion. Buffaloes/cows: 50–100 g/day.

20. *Bovimin GL (Carus Lab):* Multipurpose tonic liquid. Cows, etc. 7 ml/cow/day.
21. *Bovimin B (Carus Lab):* Multipurpose + nickel. Cows, etc. 40 g up to 10 litre milk daily; 60 g/per 20 litre milk daily; goats, etc. 20 g/day; camel 100 g/day.
22. *Latifur (Carus Lab):* Live yeast powder. Cows, etc. 1 sachet once or twice daily × 3 days.
23. *Nutrisacc bolus (Cargil):* 2 boli twice daily, orally for 15 days.
24. *Provical Forte (Cargil):* 100 ml orally, daily.
25. *HFM (Hester):* High fat, milk formula. Dose: 100 g daily.
26. *Concebov powder (Bayer):* 50–100 g/cow/day.
27. *Pecutrin powder (Bayer):* Dose 30 g/day for milk up to 20 litres or Swine: 1–2 kg/tonne of feed improves milking ability, natural resistance, and bone condition.
28. *Buff Flow powder (Bayer):* Buffaloes: 50–100 g/day for early lactation.
29. *Galactin galactogogue (Himalaya):* 4–6 boli/day/postcalving for 10 days.
30. *Himcal tonic (Himalaya):* Cow 100 ml/day; sheep/goat 40 ml daily; good for bones.
31. *Lact yeast (Neospark):* Improves immune status, digestion, and productivity; eliminates pathogenic bacteria. Dosage: Cows and Buffaloes 1 feed cake per day.
    Calves, sheep and goat ½ feed cake per day.
32. *Xtra-lac (Neospark):* Has calcium and nutrients; helps milk production, digestion, improves immunity. Dose: adult cattle and buffaloes: 60 gm per animal per day for 2–3 days.

■ ANTIFUNGAL AND ANTIDANDRUF DRUGS

1. *Dermachlor (Vetoquinol):* Medicated spray for skin (100 ml). Contains miconazole nitrate, chlorhexidine gluconate (2 % each).
   Treatment: Staphylococcus intermedius, Malassezia pachydermis, Microsporum canis, Microsporum gypsum, Trichophyton menta.
2. *Wokazole (Vetoquinol):* Miconazole, ofloxacin clobetasole, and $ZnSO_4$. 3 and 100 ml bottle. Apply lotion in mixed infections, pruritis, dermatitis, alopecia, otitis exterma, pyoderna and surgery or wounds.
3. *Kiskin cream and lotion (Intas):* Contains clobetasol propionate 0.025% w/w, ofloxacin 0.1% w/w, iconazole nitrate 2.0% w/w, zinc sulphate 3.0% w/w. Used for eczema, fungal and yeast infections, pyoderma, and allergic dermatitis. Tube of 20 g and 50 g; lotion of 30 and 100 ml.
4. *Dospray (Merial):* Spray (100 ml) containing gammabenzene hexachloride, proflavine hemisulphate, cetrimide, neem, eucalyptus oil, etc. for fungal skin infections, ringworm, yolk gall, scabies, foot rot, dognela disease, and wounds. Spray 2–3 times a day.
5. *Clinar M (Virbac):* Shampoo containing miconazole and cypermethrin. It is dual purpose shampoo. Kills fungi and skin parasites, mites and ticks.
6. *Ketochlor liquid shampoo (Virbac):* For bacterial and fungal dermatitis in dogs and cats. Wet hair coat with warm water, apply shampoo for 5–10 minutes and wash.
7. *Topicure Plus:* For wounds, FMD, dermatomycosis. Spray after shaking well.
8. *Sheen Kleen Forte:* Antifungal and antibacterial pets' shampoo. Wet hair, apply for 7–10 minutes and wash.

■ DRUGS FOR ENERGY, NEGATIVE ENERGY BALANCE, HYPOTHERMIA AND RECUMBANCY

1. *Anabolite (Virbac):* Instant energy + nicotinamide. Gluconeogenic precursors with B-complex vitamins and minerals. 1 litre pack. Dose: Cattle 100–200 ml daily.
2. *Metabolite (Virbac):* Nutritional supplement for late pregnancy. Dose: cow, etc. 100 g daily.
3. *Rintose (Vetoquinol):* Multi electrolyte and dextrose IV infusion for dehydration, diarrhoea, debility, hypoglycaemia, septicaemia, disturbed electrolyte balance, muscular weakness, systemic acidosis. Dose: Cattle, buffalo and horse: 500–2000 ml/day for 3–4 days; Sheep and goat: 100–200 ml/day for 2–3 days; Calf: 100–500 ml/day for 2–3 days; In Systemic Acidosis: Cattle & Buffalo: 1000–2000 ml/day.
4. *Woktrose (Vetoquinol):* Dextrose infusion for hypoglycaemia, ketosis, debility, emaciation, weakness, loss of appetite. Slow IV or SC injection. Warm bottle before use. Large animal 540 ml; sheep and goat: 10–150 ml; small: 25–50 ml.
5. *Klutch (Cargil):* Glucose, amino acids and protein hydrolysate powder, 1 kg packet. Dose: 50–100 g/day.
6. *Glucaboost (Natural Remedies):* Energy booster; oral. Dose: cattle, etc. 200 ml orally, daily; sheep/goats 20–30 ml/day.
7. *Intalyte (Intas):* Contains Dextrose 20% + minerals for dehydration. Packing: 500 ml and 1 litre. Dose: Cattle, etc. 200 ml, twide daily followed by 100 ml twice daily.
8. *Mifex (Novartis):* 40 ml injection. For the treatment of milk fever or associated deficiencies of magnesium and phosphrous. Mifex offers calcium, magnesium and phosphrous to meet the normal requirement of the lactating cow. Dextrose in Mifex helps maintain protein and carbohydrate metabolism during lactation and combats acetonemia. Dose: Sheep 25–75 ml.
Cattle: 200–350 ml; Administration SC or IV. Mifex oral—1 litre: dose: 500 ml twice a day.
9. *Calborol injection (Novartis):* 450 ml injection. Calborol is indicated in acute and chronic hypocalcaemia in cows, ewes, sows and bitches, is highly effective in trating milk fever with instant results, can also be used in lactation tetany to supplement injections of magnesium sulphate and in the prevention and treatment of liver damage due to chloroform or carbon tetrachloride. Slow IV injection. Dose: Canine: 2–5 ml; Sheep and Goats: 60 ml; Cattle and Horses: 200–350 ml.

■ BLEEDING PREVENTION

Jagdale Lifesciences, 782, JP Nagar, Bangalore 560078.

Clotase injection: Usable in thrombocytopenia, haemogalactia, abortion, delivery, Ehrlichiosis, dehorning, haemorrhagic gastroenteritis.

Haemogalactia: 2 ml/day for 2 days, IM/IV or 1 ml clotase diluted in 10 ml saline administered by intramammary route.

Horn amputation: 3 ml IM, then every 4–6 hours.

Before surgery: 1 ml IM/IV.

Canine haemorrhagic gastroenteritis (Bloody diarrhoea): 1 ml or 2 ml IV or IM injection. Repeat 4–6 hours.

Bovine delivery cases: 2 ml IM or IV.

Wounds of suturing: Put 1/2 to 1 vial by diluting the wounds with forceps between two sutures.

Packing: 10 ml vial.

SEPTICAEMIA

Septicaemia is common in calves, sheep and goats. My drugs of first choice are:

a. Cobactan injection—(MSD product). If covers very broad range of septicaemia producing organisms such as *P. muftaeida*, *Mannheimia*, Seph. necrophonus (foot rot) *E. coli* septicaemia (most common in calves), Staphylococci, Streptococci. Available as 50 ml vial, Dose: 2 ml per 50 kg BW by IM injection.

b. M. ceft injection (ceftriaxone injection) of Alembic. A single injection is good enough since if acts for about 96 hours (4 days) (available as vials of 1.5; 2.5 and 5 g). Dose is 5 mg per kg body weight by IV rate. In chronic cases repeat after 72 hours.

COMPLICATED FEBRILE DISEASES

In complicated febrile diseases such as contagious caprine pleuro pneumonia (CCPP), PPR, gastrointestinal infections, skin infections, aerobic and anaerobic infections (tail gangrene, dognela disease) "Floserm" (levofloxacin, 100 mg per ml) a product of Kepler is good. It is available in 100 ml pack. Inject 8 to 10 mg/kg BW by IM or IV route. It reaches peak in 1 hour. Give daily, with 98% success in bacterial diseases (breaks DNA by DNA gyrase.

Also we can use ceftriaxone and Salbactum injection (such as Ceftrivan injection of Van Vat; Safevet Forte of Merial Co/Dosch Animal Health).

Subject Index